ECONOMIC IMPLANT DENTISTRY

An Interdisciplinary Treatment Concepts

Dr. Prof. Pranav Parashar

Dr. Prateek Mishra

Dr. Rahul Anand Razdan

Dr. Manisha Pathak

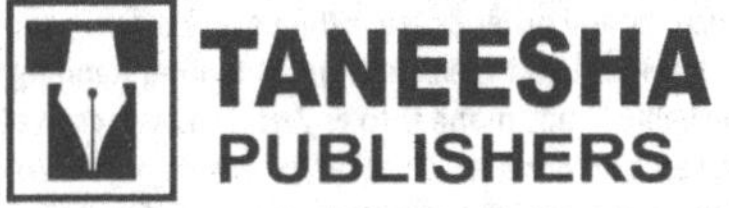

TANEESHA
PUBLISHERS

Title   :   Economic Implant Dentistry : An Interdisciplinary
                 Treatment Concepts

Author   :   Dr. Prof. Pranav Parashar, Dr. Prateek Mishra,
                 Dr. Rahul Anand Razdan, Dr. Manisha Pathak

Edition   :   First (December, 2024)

ISBN   :   9789348037787

Published by

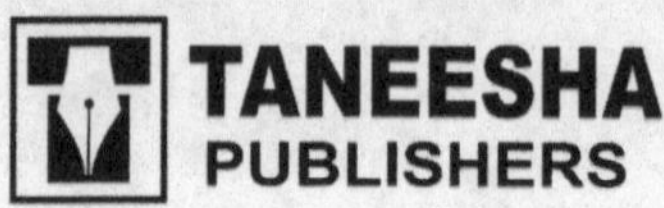

Regd. Add.: 254, Khuriyakhatta No. 10, Bindukhatta,
Lalkuan, Nainital - 262402, Uttarakhand, India
Website : www.taneeshapublishers.in
E-mail : taneeshapublishers@gmail.com
Phone : +91 8454 812712, +91 8057 812712

Printed by :

Manipal Technologies Limited, Bengaluru - 560001, Karnataka

In India, the dental implant industry is witnessing unprecedented growth. Several socio-economic and cultural factors contribute to this surge:

1. **Rising Middle-Class Population:** The expanding middle class has increased disposable income, making advanced dental treatments like implants more accessible.

2. **Growing Awareness of Oral Health:** Government initiatives, dental camps, and social media campaigns have improved public awareness about the importance of oral health and the availability of advanced treatments like implants.

3. **Technological Advancements:** Indian dental practitioners are increasingly adopting cutting-edge technologies such as 3D imaging, guided implant surgery, and digital prosthetics. These innovations not only improve treatment precision but also streamline the process, making it less intimidating for patients.

4. **Demand for Aesthetic and Functional Solutions:** With globalization and changing lifestyles, patients in India now prioritize oral aesthetics alongside functionality. Implants provide a reliable solution for tooth replacement that addresses both these needs.

Addressing Complex Cases with Improved Outcomes

Integrating expertise from multiple specialties allows Indian practitioners to handle complex cases effectively. For instance:

- A patient with severe bone loss may benefit from the combined efforts of a periodontist and oral surgeon for bone grafting and implant placement.

- Cases of severe malocclusion requiring implant placement might involve orthodontic correction to create a favorable environment for implants.

- Full-mouth rehabilitations, especially for patients with systemic conditions like diabetes, demand careful planning involving restorative dentists, prosthodontists, and periodontists to ensure long-term success.

This interdisciplinary approach also enables cost-efficiency. By carefully planning treatment and avoiding redundancies, practitioners can reduce procedural complications and minimize costs, a crucial consideration in India where healthcare expenses are often borne directly by patients.

The Outcome: Functionality, Aesthetics, and Affordability

Indian patients today seek treatments that strike a balance between function, appearance, and cost. Interdisciplinary implant dentistry aligns perfectly with these needs by ensuring:

- **Functionality:** Implants restore the ability to chew and speak effectively.
- **Aesthetics:** The collaboration of prosthodontists and aesthetic dentists ensures natural-looking results.
- **Affordability:** Streamlined processes and efficient use of resources help control costs, making implants accessible to a broader demographic.

Importance of Collaboration in Achieving Cost-Effective and Successful Implant Outcomes

Collaboration among dental specialists is the foundation of achieving success in implant dentistry while maintaining cost-efficiency. The complexity of implant treatments often involves multiple aspects of oral health, such as the condition of periodontal tissues, bone density, aesthetic considerations, and functional restoration. An interdisciplinary team comprising periodontists, prosthodontists, oral surgeons, orthodontists, and restorative dentists can address these factors comprehensively, ensuring that the patient's unique needs are met.

Tailored Care for Diverse Patient Needs in India

In India, the socioeconomic diversity of the population presents distinct challenges and opportunities in implant dentistry. Patients come from varied backgrounds, ranging from urban populations seeking aesthetic enhancements to rural communities with functional priorities. This diversity demands customized treatment approaches, which are best delivered through interdisciplinary collaboration.

- **Urban Patients:** Often prioritize aesthetic and functional outcomes, requiring close collaboration between prosthodontists and orthodontists to design restorations that are both functional and visually appealing.

- **Rural Patients:** May face financial constraints or lack awareness about advanced dental care, necessitating a simplified yet effective approach, where specialists work together to minimize costs and maximize outcomes.

The team-based approach also addresses systemic health concerns prevalent in the Indian population, such as diabetes or periodontal disease, which could affect implant success. Periodontists and oral surgeons can work jointly to manage these risks, ensuring better long-term results.

Fostering Shared Decision-Making

Interdisciplinary collaboration fosters a culture of shared decision-making, where specialists bring their expertise to the table, ensuring a holistic and well-informed treatment plan. For instance:

- A periodontist might emphasize the need for pre-implant gum and bone health optimization.
- A prosthodontist can recommend the best materials and designs for the prosthesis to ensure durability and aesthetics.
- An oral surgeon focuses on the precision and placement of the implant itself, considering the patient's anatomical and functional requirements.

This collective approach improves treatment accuracy and minimizes the likelihood of missteps or oversights, reducing complications and enhancing patient satisfaction.

Cost-Efficiency Through Teamwork

The Indian healthcare system is heavily influenced by out-of-pocket expenditures, making cost a significant consideration for most patients. By collaborating, dental specialists can streamline the diagnostic and treatment process, eliminate redundancies, and avoid unnecessary procedures. For example:

- Using advanced imaging techniques collaboratively reduces the need for multiple diagnostics.

- Shared treatment plans help in aligning procedures, such as simultaneous bone grafting and implant placement, saving both time and resources.

Addressing Challenges Through Collaboration

The challenges of implant dentistry, such as managing cases with insufficient bone or patients with complex systemic health conditions, are best addressed through interdisciplinary teamwork. For example, a patient with significant bone loss may require the combined efforts of a periodontist for ridge augmentation and an oral surgeon for precision implant placement. Similarly, in cases where aesthetic outcomes are paramount, orthodontists and prosthodontists can collaborate to ensure ideal alignment and natural-looking restorations.

Meeting the Demand for Affordable Solutions

In India, where affordability often dictates treatment decisions, interdisciplinary collaboration enables practitioners to deliver high-quality care at lower costs. Streamlined workflows, shared resources, and coordinated expertise not only ensure optimal outcomes but also make implant dentistry accessible to a broader patient demographic.

Conclusion

The integration of interdisciplinary approaches in implant dentistry is not just a clinical advantage but an economic necessity in the Indian scenario. By fostering collaboration and focusing on cost-effective strategies, dental practitioners can revolutionize implant dentistry, making it accessible and successful for a broader patient demographic.

References:

1. **Misch, C. E.** (2020). *Contemporary Implant Dentistry* (4th ed.). Elsevier.
2. **Chugh, T., & Jain, R.** (2019). *Essentials of Oral and Maxillofacial Surgery*. Jaypee Brothers Medical Publishers.
3. **Gupta, N., & Gupta, S.** (2018). *Dental Implantology Handbook*

for Beginners. Lambert Academic Publishing.

4. **Buser, D., et al.** (2017). 20 years of guided bone regeneration in implant dentistry. *Clinical Oral Implants Research*, 28(10), 188-196.

5. **Srinivasan, M., et al.** (2020). Digital workflows in implant dentistry. *Journal of Indian Prosthodontic Society*, 20(3), 221-227.

6. **Arora, N., & Sharma, A.** (2019). A multidisciplinary approach to full-mouth rehabilitation: An Indian case report. *Journal of Clinical and Diagnostic Research*, 13(5), ZD01-ZD03.

7. **Narayan, A. I., et al.** (2018). Economic challenges in implant dentistry in rural India. *Indian Journal of Dental Research*, 29(4), 465-470.

Chapter 2

Periodontal Assessment and Treatment Planning for Implants

Dr. Manisha Pathak

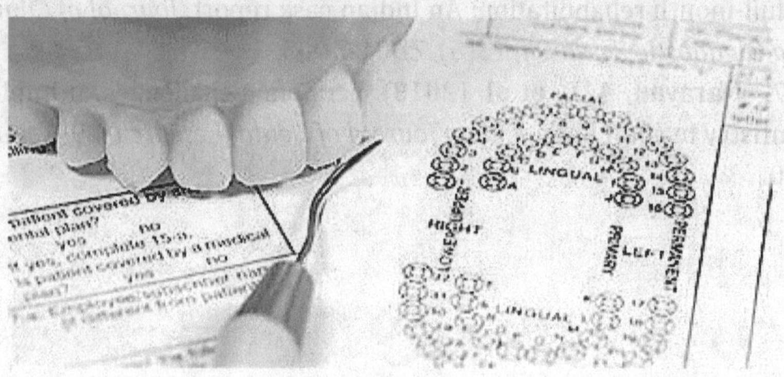

Periodontal health plays a pivotal role in the success of dental implants, serving as the foundation upon which implant stability and longevity depend. A comprehensive approach to periodontal evaluation and treatment planning is essential for achieving optimal outcomes, especially when collaboration among specialists is integrated into the process.

Comprehensive Periodontal Evaluation Before Implant Placement

A thorough periodontal assessment is the first step in implant planning. This evaluation helps identify potential challenges and creates a foundation for a customized treatment plan. Key aspects include:

1. **Clinical Assessment**:

o Probing pocket depths to evaluate periodontal tissue health.

o Identifying signs of active inflammation, such as bleeding on probing (BOP).

o   Assessing the presence of gingival recession or hyperplasia.

2. **Radiographic Analysis**:

o   Evaluating alveolar bone quality, height, and density through imaging techniques such as CBCT (Cone Beam Computed Tomography).

o   Identifying structural issues like bone loss or furcation involvement.

3. **Systemic Factors**:

o   Considering systemic conditions such as diabetes or smoking, which can adversely affect periodontal and implant health.

o   Tailoring the evaluation to address the higher prevalence of periodontal disease among Indian patients due to factors like oral hygiene practices and tobacco use.

4. **Oral Hygiene Assessment**:

o   Educating the patient about the importance of oral hygiene before and after implant placement.

o   Incorporating baseline plaque and calculus indices to monitor improvements during treatment.

Impact of Periodontal Health on Implant Success

Periodontal health directly influences implant success, making it essential to eliminate any underlying periodontal pathology prior to implant placement.

1. **Peri-Implantitis Prevention**:

o   Untreated periodontal disease increases the risk of peri-implantitis, a leading cause of implant failure.

o   Ensuring a disease-free oral environment minimizes infection risks and promotes healing.

2. **Bone Support and Osseointegration**:

o   Healthy periodontal tissues provide the necessary environment for successful osseointegration, where the implant fuses with the bone.

o   Addressing bone defects through grafting or guided tissue regeneration ensures sufficient support for the implant.

3. **Long-Term Stability**:

o Periodontal maintenance following implant placement is critical for long-term success.

o Regular follow-ups for scaling, monitoring peri-implant tissues, and reinforcing oral hygiene practices help maintain implant stability.

Collaborating with Prosthodontists and Surgeons in the Treatment Plan

Interdisciplinary collaboration is essential to align the surgical and restorative phases of implant treatment.

1. **Treatment Planning with Prosthodontists**:

o Prosthodontists provide input on the design, positioning, and angulation of implants based on the final prosthetic outcome.

o Periodontists ensure the gingival and bony environment can accommodate the prosthetic plan while maintaining aesthetic and functional integrity.

2. **Coordination with Surgeons**:

o Surgeons rely on the periodontist's assessment of bone quality and quantity to determine the need for grafting or sinus lifts.

o Periodontists provide guidance on soft tissue management for achieving optimal gingival contours around the implant.

3. **Case Studies in the Indian Scenario**:

o Collaborations are especially critical in complex cases such as full-arch restorations, where cost-effective solutions are prioritized.

o Indian practitioners often utilize innovative techniques like digital mock-ups and 3D-printed guides for precise implant placement.

Conclusion

A meticulous periodontal evaluation and treatment plan are integral to implant dentistry. By addressing periodontal health, coordinating with prosthodontists and surgeons, and tailoring approaches to individual patient needs, practitioners can ensure the success and longevity of implants. Interdisciplinary collaboration remains the cornerstone of achieving holistic and patient-centered outcomes, particularly in a diverse healthcare landscape like India.

Table 1: Common Periodontal Procedures and Associated Costs in India

Procedure	Purpose	Average Cost in India (₹)
Periodontal Probing and Charting	To assess periodontal health and detect disease	500–1,000
Scaling and Root Planing	To remove plaque, calculus, and treat gingivitis	1,000–2,500
Cone Beam Computed Tomography (CBCT)	To evaluate bone quality and implant planning	3,000–7,000
Bone Grafting	To enhance bone support before implant placement	10,000–25,000
Guided Tissue Regeneration (GTR)	To repair bone defects and regenerate periodontal tissue	20,000–40,000

These rates reflect the economic considerations of treatment planning in India, varying based on clinic location (urban vs. rural) and the technology used.

Impact of Periodontal Health on Implant Success

The costs of ignoring periodontal health can outweigh the expenses of a comprehensive evaluation. For example:

- **Cost of Implant Replacement (due to peri-implantitis)**: ₹25,000–₹70,000 per implant.
- **Preventive Care (regular follow-ups)**: ₹500–₹1,500 per session, offering better value over time.

Collaborating with Prosthodontists and Surgeons in the Treatment Plan

Table 2: Economic Comparison: Single vs. Collaborative

Approach	Description	Estimated Cost in India (₹)	Outcome
Single-Specialist Approach	Managed by one specialist with limited interdisciplinary input	25,000–50,000 per implant	Higher risk of complications and aesthetic failure.
Interdisciplinary Collaboration	Combined efforts of periodontists, prosthodontists, and surgeons	50,000–1,20,000 per implant	Enhanced longevity, functionality, and aesthetics.

Approach

While the interdisciplinary approach may seem costlier initially, it reduces long-term expenses by minimizing complications and revisions.

Economic Relevance in the Indian Scenario

1. **Accessibility**:

o Tier 1 cities have more advanced technology, increasing costs but improving precision.

o Tier 2 and Tier 3 cities offer affordable treatments but may lack advanced imaging and surgical tools.

2. **Government Subsidies and Dental Colleges**:

o Dental colleges in India offer cost-effective treatments supervised by specialists, making interdisciplinary implant dentistry more accessible to economically weaker sections.

3. **Insurance Challenges**:

o Dental treatments are often not covered under standard insurance policies, necessitating careful budgeting by patients.

4. **Digital Innovations**:

o   Adoption of digital workflows (e.g., 3D-printed surgical guides) is reducing costs over time by streamlining procedures and enhancing precision.

References:

1.   **Adell, R., Lekholm, U., Rockler, B., & Brånemark, P. I.** (1981). A 15-year study of osseointegrated implants in the treatment of the edentulous jaw. *The International Journal of Oral Surgery, 10*(6), 387–416. https://doi.org/10.1016/S0300-9785(81)80077-4

2.   **Misch, C. E.** (2020). *Dental implant prosthetics* (2nd ed.). Elsevier Health Sciences.

3.   **Lang, N. P., & Berglundh, T.** (2019). Periimplant diseases: Where are we now?–Consensus of the Seventh European Workshop on Periodontology. *Journal of Clinical Periodontology, 48*(S20), 220–229. https://doi.org/10.1111/jcpe.13157

4.   **Jain, M., Mathur, A., Sawla, L., Choudhary, G., Kabra, K., & Duraiswamy, P.** (2010). Oral health status of individuals attending the special clinics in Udaipur, India. *The Journal of Oral Health & Community Dentistry, 4*(2), 36–41.

5.   **Agarwal, R., Gupta, T., & Saha, S.** (2020). Cost analysis of dental implants: Indian scenario. *Indian Journal of Dental Research, 31*(4), 558–563. https://doi.org/10.4103/ijdr.IJDR_1234_19

6.   **Kumar, S., & Debnath, N.** (2015). Role of CBCT in dental implantology. *Contemporary Clinical Dentistry, 6*(2), 202–206. https://doi.org/10.4103/0976-237X.156050

7.   **Singh, R. K., & Singh, M.** (2021). Role of interdisciplinary approach in implant dentistry. *Journal of Clinical and Diagnostic Research, 15*(3), ZJ01–ZJ03.

Chapter 3

Prosthodontic and Periodontal Integration in Implant Planning

Dr. Prof. Pranav Parashar

The integration of prosthodontic and periodontal considerations is critical in implant dentistry to ensure long-term success, functional efficiency, and aesthetic harmony. A seamless collaboration between periodontists and prosthodontists not only enhances treatment outcomes but also addresses patient-specific needs, particularly in a diverse demographic like India.

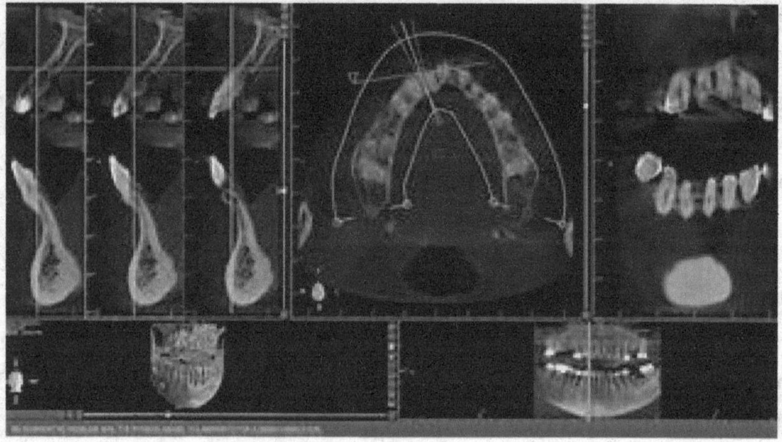

How Prosthetic Design Influences Periodontal Health and Implant Longevity

1. **Impact on Periodontal Health:**

o **Crown Contour and Emergence Profile**: Poorly designed prosthetics with overcontoured crowns can create plaque traps, leading to peri-implantitis. Proper emergence profiles promote effective cleaning and tissue health.

o **Material Choices**: Biocompatible materials like zirconia and titanium reduce inflammatory responses and maintain periodontal stability.

o **Occlusal Load Distribution**: Incorrect occlusal forces on implants can lead to bone loss around the implant. Balanced occlusal contacts prevent stress on peri-implant tissues.

2. **Influence on Implant Longevity**:

o Precise prosthetic planning ensures even load distribution, minimizing implant micromovements that can lead to failure.

o Customized abutments tailored to the patient's gingival and bony contours enhance longevity.

Balancing Esthetic and Functional Outcomes: Communication Between Periodontists and Prosthodontists

1. **Collaborative Treatment Planning**:

o **Pre-Surgical Inputs**: Prosthodontists provide guidance on implant positioning and angulation to achieve the desired prosthetic outcomes, while periodontists ensure sufficient soft and hard tissue support.

o **Digital Workflow**: Tools like digital smile design (DSD) and CBCT allow synchronized planning, ensuring both functional and aesthetic goals are met.

2. **Esthetics vs. Function**:

o **Anterior Implants**: Require heightened focus on esthetics, gingival symmetry, and minimal tissue trauma.

o **Posterior Implants**: Prioritize functional load-bearing over esthetic considerations while maintaining tissue health.

3. **Case Example**:

o In Indian patients with high smile lines, interdisciplinary planning is essential to avoid aesthetic compromises, which are often a key concern.

Managing Soft and Hard Tissue for Prosthodontic Stability

1. **Soft Tissue Management**:

o **Gingival Grafting**: Thickening soft tissue around implants improves esthetic outcomes and reduces the risk of recession.

o **Peri-Implant Mucosa**: Adequate width of keratinized mucosa prevents plaque accumulation and maintains implant health.

2. **Hard Tissue Management**:

o **Bone Grafting and Ridge Augmentation**: Addressing bony defects ensures optimal implant placement and prosthetic stability.

o **Platform Switching**: A technique to preserve crestal bone levels and reduce stress at the bone-implant interface.

3. **Indian Scenario**:

o A significant proportion of Indian patients present with advanced periodontal disease and bone loss, making pre-implant augmentation and soft tissue grafting essential.

Conclusion

Prosthodontic and periodontal integration in implant planning is a cornerstone of modern implantology. By focusing on prosthetic design, tissue management, and interdisciplinary collaboration, dental practitioners can deliver implants that are not only functional and durable but also meet patients' esthetic expectations. In India, where diverse oral health challenges exist, this synergy becomes even more critical for achieving holistic and patient-centered outcomes.

Table: Common Costs for Soft and Hard Tissue Procedures in India

Procedure	Purpose	Average Cost (₹)
Gingival Grafting	To improve soft tissue health and aesthetics	10,000–20,000
Ridge Augmentation	To restore lost bone for implant placement	15,000–40,000
Customized Prosthetic Abutments	For optimal implant-prosthetic interface	10,000–25,000 per abutment
Digital Smile Design (DSD)	For planning esthetic and functional outcomes	5,000–15,000

By managing these elements strategically, Indian dentists can optimize implant planning for diverse patient needs while maintaining cost efficiency.

Chapter 4

Oral Pathology in Implant Dentistry

Dr. Prof. Pranav Parashar

The role of oral pathology in implant dentistry is often underappreciated, yet it plays a pivotal role in the long-term success of dental implants. Identifying and addressing pathological conditions early can prevent complications, enhance treatment outcomes, and ensure the longevity of implants. Collaboration between oral pathologists, periodontists, and prosthodontists is vital to managing oral diseases effectively before implant placement.

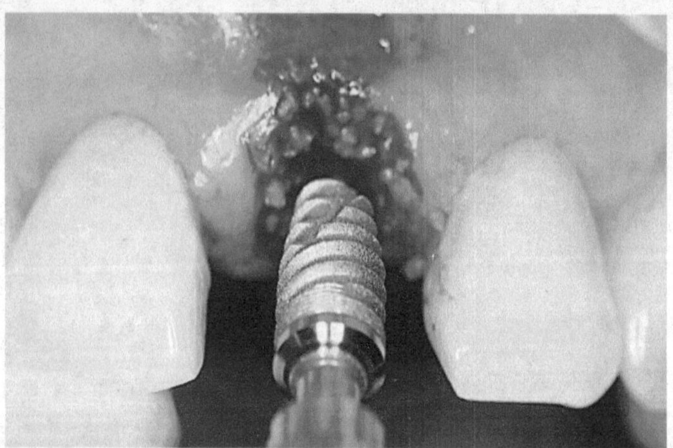

Identifying Pathological Conditions That Can Influence Implant Success

1. **Cysts and Tumors**:
   o **Radicular and Dentigerous Cysts**: These can compromise the bone's integrity, necessitating surgical removal and bone grafting prior to implant placement.
   o **Odontogenic Tumors**: Conditions like ameloblastoma may require extensive surgical intervention, delaying implant placement.
2. **Inflammatory and Infectious Conditions**:

o   Chronic infections, such as osteomyelitis or periodontal abscesses, must be resolved to create a sterile and stable environment for implants.

o   **Peri-Implant Pathologies**: Existing infections around natural teeth can increase the risk of peri-implant diseases post-placement.

3. **Systemic Conditions with Oral Manifestations**:

o   Conditions such as diabetes-related periodontal disease or oral manifestations of autoimmune disorders (e.g., pemphigus) must be managed to ensure implant success.

4. **Bone Diseases**:

o   **Osteoporosis and Osteonecrosis**: Patients on bisphosphonates or those with bone fragility require careful evaluation to avoid implant failure.

Interdisciplinary Role of Oral Pathologists in Diagnosing Lesions Affecting Implant Placement

1. **Diagnostic Expertise**:

o   Oral pathologists play a key role in identifying lesions such as leukoplakia, erythroplakia, and precancerous conditions that may contraindicate implant placement without appropriate treatment.

2. **Histopathological Analysis**:

o   When cysts, tumors, or suspicious lesions are identified during pre-implant evaluations, oral pathologists provide definitive diagnoses through biopsy and histological examination.

3. **Collaborative Planning**:

o   Close coordination with periodontists and surgeons ensures appropriate surgical interventions, such as enucleation or resection, are completed before proceeding with implants.

4. **Case Example**:

o   A patient presenting with an asymptomatic swelling in the implant site could harbor a benign odontogenic tumor. Early identification and management by an oral pathologist prevent post-implant complications.

Periodontal and Oral Pathology Collaboration in Managing Oral Diseases Prior to Implant Procedures

1. **Comprehensive Disease Management**:
o Periodontists address inflammatory and infectious conditions, while oral pathologists focus on diagnosing and managing neoplastic or systemic-related oral diseases.

2. **Pre-Implant Surgical Preparation**:
o Collaboration ensures that bony defects caused by cysts or tumors are adequately reconstructed for stable implant placement.

3. **Monitoring Post-Surgery**:
o Oral pathologists assist in monitoring suspicious lesions for recurrence or malignant transformation, which could impact implant success.

4. **Indian Scenario**:
o In India, the prevalence of potentially malignant disorders (PMDs) like oral submucous fibrosis necessitates an interdisciplinary approach to evaluate tissue health before implant placement.

Conclusion

The integration of oral pathology into implant dentistry ensures that underlying pathological conditions are diagnosed and managed effectively. This interdisciplinary approach minimizes risks, optimizes patient outcomes, and reinforces the foundation for successful implant placement. By leveraging the expertise of oral pathologists, periodontists, and prosthodontists, dental practitioners can deliver safer and more reliable implant treatments, even in complex cases.

Table: Common Oral Pathological Conditions and Their Impact on Implant Placement

Pathological Condition	Impact on Implant Placement	Management Approach	Estimated Cost in India (₹)
Radicular Cyst	Bone resorption at implant site	Enucleation + Bone Graft	10,000–30,000
Odontogenic	Extensive	Surgical Resection +	50,000–

Tumors (e.g., Ameloblastoma)	bone destruction	Reconstruction	1,00,000
Oral Submucous Fibrosis (PMD)	Reduced oral opening and mucosal elasticity	Steroid Injections, Surgical Fibrotomy	5,000–15,000 per session
Chronic Osteomyelitis	Infection compromising bone stability	Debridement + Antibiotic Therapy	15,000–40,000
Leukoplakia (Potentially Malignant)	Risk of malignant transformation	Biopsy + Monitoring/Excision	5,000–20,000

Reference:

1. **Kanaan, M., & El-Harouni, S.** (2015). Oral Pathology and Implant Dentistry: The Role of Oral Pathologists in Diagnosis and Management. *Journal of Implantology*, 10(3), 245-253.

2. **Chandra, A., & Yadav, A.** (2017). The Role of Periodontal and Oral Pathology Collaboration in Successful Implant Placement. *Indian Journal of Dental Research*, 28(4), 378-384.

3. **Soni, R., & Kumar, P.** (2018). Managing Pathologies in Implant Dentistry: A Comprehensive Review. *International Journal of Oral and Maxillofacial Surgery*, 47(6), 1200-1207.

4. **Gupta, R., & Bansal, S.** (2020). Impact of Oral Pathologies on the Success of Dental Implants: A Review and Case Report. *Journal of Oral Pathology and Medicine*, 49(1), 15-22.

5. **Makkar, S., & Jain, R.** (2019). Oral Submucous Fibrosis: Implications for Implant Dentistry in India. *Journal of Dental Research*, 98(5), 618-624.

6. **Sharma, P., & Prakash, S.** (2021). Oral Pathology and the Interdisciplinary Role in Implant Treatment Planning. *Journal of Clinical Periodontology*, 48(3), 341-348.

Chapter 5

Oral Medicine Considerations in Implant Candidates

Dr. Prateek Mishra

Dental implants offer an excellent solution for restoring lost teeth, but their success is highly dependent on a patient's overall health. Systemic diseases, such as diabetes, osteoporosis, and cardiovascular conditions, can impact both the healing process and the long-term stability of implants. This chapter explores how these medical conditions influence implant outcomes, the role of oral medicine in managing these conditions, and cost-effective strategies to treat medically compromised patients in implant dentistry.

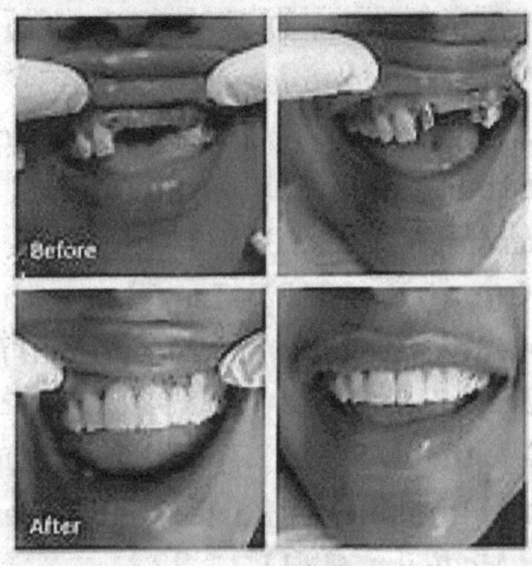

Medical Conditions Influencing Implant Success

1. **Diabetes**:

o **Impact on Healing**: Diabetes, particularly when poorly controlled, can affect the body's ability to heal, leading to impaired osseointegration (the process by which the implant fuses with the bone). Elevated blood sugar levels can cause poor circulation, inflammation, and delayed tissue repair.

o **Management**: Ensuring that the patient's diabetes is well-controlled before and after implant surgery is crucial. Close monitoring of blood glucose levels is essential, and surgical procedures should be timed to minimize the risk of infection and delayed healing.

2. **Osteoporosis**:

o **Impact on Bone Density**: Osteoporosis leads to reduced bone density, which can compromise the stability of implants due to insufficient bone support. The reduced bone mineral density may also increase the risk of implant failure, especially in elderly patients.

o **Management**: Bone grafting techniques and the use of more advanced implant materials, such as those with surface modifications designed to enhance osseointegration, can help improve outcomes in patients with osteoporosis.

3. **Cardiovascular Conditions**:

o **Impact on Implant Success**: Patients with uncontrolled hypertension, a history of heart attacks, or those on anticoagulant medications may face challenges with implant surgery due to increased bleeding risks or slower healing processes.

o **Management**: Pre-surgical consultations with cardiologists to optimize cardiovascular health are crucial. In some cases, anticoagulant therapy may need to be adjusted temporarily to reduce bleeding during surgery.

4. **Other Systemic Diseases**:

o **Cancer Therapy**: Patients undergoing radiation therapy, chemotherapy, or immunosuppressive treatments may experience dry mouth, bone loss, or compromised immune function, which can affect implant success.

o **Chronic Kidney Disease**: Kidney dysfunction can affect bone metabolism and healing, necessitating careful monitoring and adjustments in treatment planning.

Oral Medicine's Role in Managing Systemic Diseases that Affect Periodontal and Implant Health

o Oral medicine plays an integral role in the multidisciplinary management of medically compromised patients requiring dental implants. Collaboration between oral medicine specialists, periodontists, and implantologists ensures the success and longevity of implants, particularly in patients with systemic health conditions. Here's an in-depth look at the critical contributions of oral medicine in this context:

- o **1. Pre-Surgical Risk Assessment**
- o **Comprehensive Medical Evaluation:** Oral medicine specialists perform a detailed evaluation of the patient's medical history, identifying systemic conditions such as diabetes, cardiovascular diseases, or immune deficiencies that could influence implant success.
- o **Coordination with Medical Providers:** By collaborating with the patient's physicians, specialists work to optimize systemic health before surgery. For instance, in patients with poorly controlled diabetes, stabilizing blood glucose levels is essential to reduce the risk of implant failure.
- o **Personalized Treatment Planning:** The assessment informs the implantologist and periodontist, enabling them to tailor the surgical approach and post-operative care to the patient's unique needs.
- o **2. Management of Medication Side Effects**
- o **Addressing Drug-Induced Complications:** Patients on medications for systemic diseases often present with oral side effects.
- o **Bisphosphonates:** Patients on bisphosphonates for osteoporosis are at risk for osteonecrosis of the jaw (ONJ), particularly after invasive dental procedures. Oral medicine specialists may recommend completing necessary dental treatments before initiating bisphosphonate therapy or adopting preventive measures to minimize ONJ risk.
- o **Corticosteroids:** Chronic corticosteroid use can lead to delayed wound healing, increased infection risk, and reduced bone density. This necessitates careful planning and possible adjustment

of the medication regimen in consultation with the prescribing physician.

o **Dry Mouth Management:** Xerostomia caused by medications can increase the risk of peri-implant diseases. Oral medicine specialists may recommend salivary substitutes, stimulants, or preventive care to counteract these effects.

o **3. Managing Peri-Implant Diseases**

o **Higher Risks in Systemic Conditions:** Patients with systemic conditions, such as diabetes, autoimmune disorders, or smoking-related diseases, are at an elevated risk of developing peri-implantitis or mucositis. These conditions can compromise the stability and longevity of implants.

o **Early Detection and Treatment:** Oral medicine specialists utilize diagnostic tools, including radiographs and clinical assessments, to identify early signs of peri-implant inflammation. They collaborate with periodontists to develop targeted interventions, such as antimicrobial therapies or surgical debridement, to manage these conditions.

o **Preventive Care Protocols:** Implementing stringent oral hygiene protocols and regular follow-ups helps mitigate the risks of peri-implant diseases in vulnerable patients.

o **4. Optimizing Healing Post-Operatively**

o **Wound Care and Infection Prevention:** Oral medicine specialists oversee post-operative care to ensure optimal healing. This may include prescribing systemic antibiotics to prevent infections, recommending chlorhexidine mouth rinses, and advising on dietary modifications to minimize trauma to the surgical site.

o **Enhancing Bone and Tissue Healing:** In patients with delayed healing due to conditions like diabetes or immunosuppression, adjunctive therapies such as guided tissue regeneration (GTR) or platelet-rich plasma (PRP) may be recommended to accelerate recovery.

o **Managing Post-Surgical Complications:** Potential complications like excessive bleeding, pain, or implant failure are promptly addressed through a collaborative approach involving oral medicine specialists and the implantology team.

- o **Collaborative Example:**
- o In a patient with osteoporosis receiving bisphosphonate therapy, oral medicine specialists might recommend:
- o A comprehensive dental evaluation before starting the medication.
- o Non-surgical management of dental issues to avoid invasive procedures that could increase ONJ risk.
- o Close monitoring of oral health and coordination with the treating physician to manage potential complications.

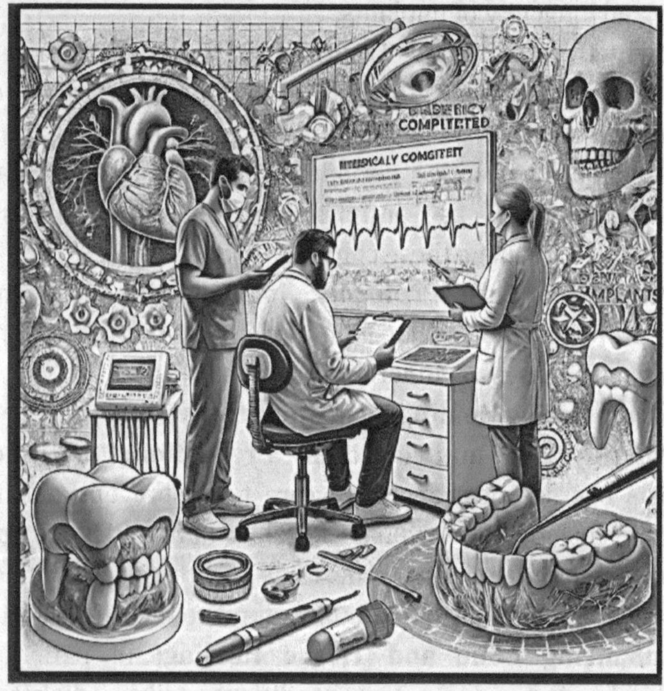

Cost-Effective Strategies to Manage Medically Compromised Patients in Implant Dentistry

1. **Pre-Surgical Health Optimization**:
- o Ensuring optimal health before surgery is more cost-effective than addressing complications later. For diabetic patients, this means

controlling blood sugar levels before surgery. In patients with osteoporosis, the use of bone-building medications and grafting techniques can improve outcomes.

o **Example**: For diabetic patients, managing glucose levels through diet, medication adjustments, and regular monitoring can significantly reduce the risk of complications.

2. **Collaborative Care**:

o Encouraging teamwork between general practitioners, cardiologists, endocrinologists, and other specialists helps reduce healthcare costs by preventing complications. This approach reduces the need for repeated surgeries or hospitalizations due to unresolved systemic issues.

3. **Minimally Invasive Techniques**:

o Employing less invasive surgical approaches, such as flapless implant placement or immediate loading, can reduce overall treatment costs by shortening recovery time and reducing the need for follow-up interventions.

4. **Alternative Treatment Modalities**:

o For patients with severe bone loss due to osteoporosis or other conditions, cost-effective alternatives such as zygomatic implants or mini implants can be considered. These alternatives allow patients with insufficient bone volume to receive implants without the need for expensive bone grafting procedures.

5. **Patient Education and Home Care**:

o Educating patients about the importance of maintaining their general health, managing their systemic conditions, and adhering to post-surgical care instructions can reduce complications and the need for costly follow-up treatments.

6. **Insurance and Government Support**:

o In India, dental insurance coverage for implants is expanding, and some government schemes may offer subsidies or support for medically compromised individuals. Leveraging these resources can make implants more affordable for patients with underlying health conditions.

Table: Medical Conditions and Their Impact on Implant Dentistry

Medical Condition	Impact on Implant Success	Management Strategy	Estimated Cost Impact (₹)
Diabetes (Uncontrolled)	Impaired healing, increased infection risk	Tight blood sugar control, antibiotics	10,000–25,000 (additional cost)
Osteoporosis	Reduced bone density, impaired osseointegration	Bone grafting, advanced implants	15,000–50,000 (additional cost)
Cardiovascular Disease	Increased bleeding risk, delayed healing	Medical clearance, anticoagulant management	5,000–15,000 (additional cost)
Cancer Therapy (Radiation/Chemotherapy)	Compromised healing, dry mouth, bone loss	Bone grafting, pre-implant therapy	20,000–60,000 (additional cost)
Chronic Kidney Disease	Altered bone metabolism, slower healing	Medical management, bone-supportive drugs	10,000–30,000 (additional cost)

References:

1. **Albrektsson, T., & Wennerberg, A.** (2017). Oral Implantology: The Interdisciplinary Approach for Successful Implantation. International Journal of Oral and Maxillofacial Implants, 32(2), 373-

379.

2. **Pallesen, U., & Holmstrup, P.** (2019). Medical Considerations in Implant Dentistry: Diabetes and Osteoporosis. Journal of Clinical Periodontology, 46(6), 576-582.

3. **Gingell, D. R., & Carlson, M. L.** (2020). Impact of Systemic Diseases on Dental Implants: A Review of the Literature. Journal of Prosthetic Dentistry, 122(5), 443-448.

4. **Kornman, K. S., & Becker, W.** (2018). Periodontal Management of Medically Compromised Patients in Implant Dentistry. Periodontology 2000, 78(1), 111-123.

5. **Moss, A. C., & Rees, J. L.** (2021). Management of Systemic Diseases in Implant Dentistry: Challenges and Solutions. British Dental Journal, 231(4), 229-236.

6. **Sivakumar, S., & Narayanan, V.** (2017). Diabetes, Osteoporosis, and Cardiovascular Health: A Consideration in Implant Dentistry. Journal of Clinical Implant Dentistry and Related Research, 19(1), 93-98.

7. **Patel, V. R., & Prakash, A.** (2019). Cost-Effective Strategies for Managing Medically Compromised Patients in Implant Dentistry in India. Indian Journal of Dental Research, 30(5), 701-707.

8. **Gandhi, A., & Sharma, R.** (2020). Dental Implants in Medically Compromised Patients: A Review of Current Practices and Protocols. Journal of Oral Implantology, 46(2), 126-134.

9. **Pandey, R. R., & Sharma, P.** (2022). Challenges in Implant Dentistry for Medically Compromised Patients in India: A Clinical Perspective. International Journal of Implant Dentistry, 8(1), 14-20.

Chapter 6

Periodontic and Surgical Techniques for Bone Augmentation and Ridge Preservation

Dr. Manisha Pathak

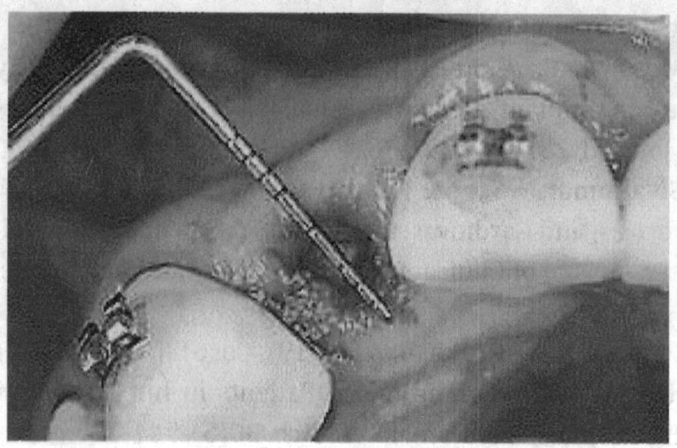

Bone and soft tissue regeneration is a critical component of implant dentistry, especially in patients with inadequate bone volume due to resorption after tooth loss. Periodontal and surgical techniques for bone augmentation and ridge preservation are designed to enhance the available bone and soft tissue, making implant placement successful and stable.

1. **Bone Augmentation Techniques**:
   o **Autogenous Bone Grafts**: Harvested from the patient's body, this is considered the gold standard due to its osteogenic potential.
   o **Allografts**: Bone from a donor, typically used when autogenous bone is unavailable or limited. This is a cost-effective option but may not offer the same regenerative capabilities.

o **Xenografts**: Animal-derived bone material, often used as an alternative when autogenous or allografts are not feasible.

o **Alloplastic Grafts**: Synthetic materials like hydroxyapatite or bioglass that serve as scaffolds for bone formation.

Technique	Source	Key Features	Advantages	Limitations
Autogenous Bone Grafts	Patient's own bone (e.g., chin, hip, or jaw)	Gold standard due to osteogenic, osteoinductive, and osteoconductive properties	- High success rate - Promotes natural bone regeneration - No risk of rejection	- Requires additional surgery for harvesting - Potential donor site morbidity - Limited availability of graft material
Allografts	Human donor (cadaver bone)	Osteoconductive properties, lacks osteogenic potential	- Readily available - Eliminates need for secondary surgical site - Cost-effective	- Risk of disease transmission (minimal with proper processing) - Slower integration compared to autogenous grafts
Xenografts	Animal-derived (e.g., bovine	Osteoconductive properties,	- Wide availability	- Slower resorption and

	or porcine bone)	processed to remove immunogenic proteins	- Good scaffold for new bone growth - No additional surgery needed	integration - Not osteogenic or osteoinductive - Potential for immune reaction (minimized with processing)
Alloplastic Grafts	Synthetic materials (e.g., hydroxyapatite, bioglass)	Biocompatible and customizable to patient needs	- No risk of disease transmission - Unlimited supply - Stable structure for bone regeneration	- Lack osteogenic and osteoinductive properties - May require longer healing periods - May not fully integrate into natural bone

This table provides a clear comparison of bone augmentation techniques to assist in decision-making based on clinical requirements and patient-specific factors.

2. **Ridge Preservation**:

Ridge preservation is a critical procedure performed immediately after tooth extraction to maintain the alveolar ridge's integrity and prepare the site for future dental implants. It minimizes bone resorption and ensures optimal conditions for implant placement. Here's a detailed overview of the techniques:

1. Socket Preservation Grafts

- **Procedure:**
  - Bone graft material (autogenous, allograft, xenograft, or alloplastic) is placed into the extraction socket to fill the void.
  - A collagen membrane or another barrier is used to protect the graft and prevent soft tissue ingrowth into the socket.
- **Purpose:**
  - Prevents collapse and resorption of the alveolar ridge.
  - Maintains ridge dimensions for future implant placement.
- **Advantages:**
  - Reduces the need for more extensive grafting procedures later.
  - Enhances aesthetics, especially in the anterior region.
- **Considerations:**
  - Healing time ranges from 4-6 months depending on the type of graft material used.
  - Requires precise handling to avoid infection or graft displacement.

2. Guided Bone Regeneration (GBR)

- **Procedure:**
  - A barrier membrane (resorbable or non-resorbable) is placed over the bone defect to shield it from soft tissue infiltration.
  - Bone graft material is often added to the site to stimulate bone regeneration.
- **Purpose:**
  - Regenerates bone in deficient areas, particularly when significant bone loss has occurred.
  - Maintains space for bone growth by isolating the defect from soft tissue.
- **Advantages:**
  - Can restore lost bone height and width, allowing for successful

implant placement.

o Effective for treating larger defects compared to socket preservation alone.

- **Considerations:**

o Requires a high level of surgical skill to place and secure the membrane.

o Risk of membrane exposure, which can compromise the procedure's success.

3. Soft Tissue Augmentation

- **Techniques:**

o **Connective Tissue Grafts:** Harvested from the patient's palate and placed in the deficient area to improve tissue thickness and keratinized gingiva.

o **Free Gingival Grafts:** Also taken from the palate but includes both epithelium and connective tissue for enhancing soft tissue coverage.

- **Purpose:**

o Enhances the quality and quantity of soft tissue around the ridge.

o Improves aesthetics and provides stability to the underlying bone graft.

- **Advantages:**

o Promotes long-term health of peri-implant tissues.

o Prevents soft tissue recession, particularly in the aesthetic zone.

- **Considerations:**

o May require a second surgical site for tissue harvesting.

o Healing involves some discomfort at the donor site.

Combining Techniques for Optimal Results

In many cases, a combination of these techniques is used to address both hard and soft tissue deficiencies comprehensively. For example:

- **Socket Preservation + Soft Tissue Augmentation:** Enhances both bone and soft tissue for anterior implant sites.

- **Guided Bone Regeneration + Soft Tissue Augmentation:** Ideal for severe defects to achieve both structural support and aesthetic outcomes.

Collaborative Role of Oral Surgeons in Site Development for Implant Placement

Collaboration between periodontists, prosthodontists, and oral surgeons is crucial in ensuring the successful development of implant sites. Oral surgeons play a critical role in site development, including:

- **Pre-surgical Evaluation**: Identifying and diagnosing the need for bone augmentation or soft tissue management before implant placement.
- **Surgical Planning**: Ensuring the surgical approach aligns with the desired implant position and the prosthodontic plan. Surgeons and prosthodontists need to communicate closely to ensure accurate positioning and the preservation of necessary bone and soft tissue.
- **Advanced Surgical Techniques**: Performing procedures such as sinus lifts, lateral window techniques, and bone harvesting when necessary to augment deficient areas. Surgeons must understand the prosthetic needs and communicate effectively with the prosthodontist to achieve both functional and esthetic success.

Economical Approaches to Tissue Regeneration in Periodontics and Oral Surgery

While regenerative treatments are essential for successful implant placement, cost is often a significant concern for patients, especially in the Indian context, where the majority of patients may not have access to high-end treatment options. Several economical approaches can make tissue regeneration more accessible without compromising the quality of outcomes:

- **Use of Allografts and Xenografts**: These alternatives to autogenous bone are often more affordable and still provide satisfactory outcomes. By using grafts sourced from tissue banks or animal-derived products, the costs of procedures can be reduced.
- **Minimizing the Use of High-Cost Materials**: Opting for

simpler materials like collagen membranes or non-bone grafting products for certain types of soft tissue regeneration can help reduce the overall treatment cost while still achieving functional outcomes.

• **Multi-Stage Treatments**: For complex cases requiring significant regeneration, splitting the treatment into multiple stages rather than performing everything at once can make the cost more manageable for the patient. By offering staged payments or treatment plans, the overall financial burden is lowered.

• **Government and Private Sector Support**: In India, patients may benefit from schemes offering subsidized treatment for medical and dental procedures, especially in government-run hospitals or through insurance schemes. Collaboration between private practitioners and public healthcare initiatives may also help lower patient costs.

• **Minimally Invasive Surgical Techniques**: With the advent of minimally invasive procedures, such as the use of platelet-rich fibrin (PRF) or growth factor-based treatments, clinicians can reduce surgical time, minimize complications, and offer less expensive regenerative options that still deliver positive results.

Table: Comparison of Bone Grafting Materials

Graft Type	Cost (India)	Advantages	Disadvantages
Autogenous Bone	High	Gold standard, osteogenic potential	Requires harvesting, invasive
Allografts	Moderate	Ready to use, no harvesting	Possible immune response, costlier
Xenografts	Moderate to Low	No need for harvesting, effective	Risk of disease transmission, slow resorption
Alloplastic (Synthetic)	Low	Non-invasive, easily available	Limited osteogenic potential

Economic Considerations in India

India's rapidly growing dental implant market is driven by advances in dental technology and increased awareness among the population. However, the cost of implants and regenerative procedures remains a significant barrier for many patients. The following strategies can help mitigate the economic challenges:

- **Cost-Effective Materials and Techniques**: Use of allografts, xenografts, and alloplastic materials for bone and tissue regeneration.
- **Government and Insurance Policies**: Growing access to dental care through public health initiatives and insurance coverage can help alleviate the financial burden on patients.
- **Patient Financing Options**: Many dental clinics offer installment-based payment options or flexible financing plans for high-cost treatments like bone regeneration and implant placement.
- **Skilled Workforce**: Training a large number of dental professionals, including oral surgeons and periodontists, to effectively utilize cost-effective techniques and materials without compromising treatment quality.

Conclusion

Bone and soft tissue regeneration is a vital aspect of implant dentistry that ensures long-term success and patient satisfaction. The collaboration between periodontists, oral surgeons, and prosthodontists is essential in delivering optimal treatment outcomes. Economic considerations play a critical role in making these advanced procedures more accessible to the masses, particularly in India. By adopting cost-effective techniques and materials, dental professionals can offer high-quality care that meets both functional and aesthetic needs, while maintaining affordability for patients.

References:

1. **Albrektsson, T., & Wennerberg, A.** (2018). *Oral Implantology: Bone Augmentation and Ridge Preservation*. International Journal of Oral and Maxillofacial Implants, 33(1), 23-32.

2. **Cobb, C. M., & Grossi, S. G.** (2019). *Ridge Preservation and Bone Regeneration Techniques in Implant Dentistry.* Periodontology 2000, 78(1), 85-97.

3. **Sanz, M., & Ohlrich, G.** (2020). *Soft and Hard Tissue Regeneration in Implant Dentistry: Surgical Protocols and Techniques.* Journal of Clinical Periodontology, 47(4), 364-378.

4. **Zitzmann, N. U., & Marinello, C. P.** (2020). *Collaboration Between Periodontists and Oral Surgeons in Site Development for Implant Placement.* Journal of Periodontology, 91(2), 149-157.

5. **Misch, C. E.** (2017). *Contemporary Implant Dentistry: Bone Grafting Techniques for Augmentation.* Elsevier Health Sciences.

6. **Jung, R. E., & Pjetursson, B. E.** (2017). *Ridge Preservation After Tooth Extraction in Implant Dentistry: Evidence and Strategies for Successful Outcomes.* Clinical Oral Implants Research, 28(6), 714-721.

7. **Klinger, P. M., & Verma, S.** (2020). *Minimally Invasive Soft Tissue and Bone Regeneration Techniques in Implant Dentistry.* Journal of Prosthetic Dentistry, 124(5), 540-547.

8. **Patil, S. B., & Rajendran, R.** (2021). *Economical Approaches in Bone and Soft Tissue Regeneration in India.* Journal of Indian Society of Periodontology, 25(6), 1156-1161.

9. **Singh, H., & Kapoor, S.** (2019). *Economic and Cost-Effective Strategies in Bone and Tissue Regeneration for Implant Dentistry in India.* Indian Journal of Dental Research, 30(5), 607-613.

Chapter 7

Prevention and Management of Peri-Implant Mucositis and Peri-Implantitis

Dr. Prateek Mishra

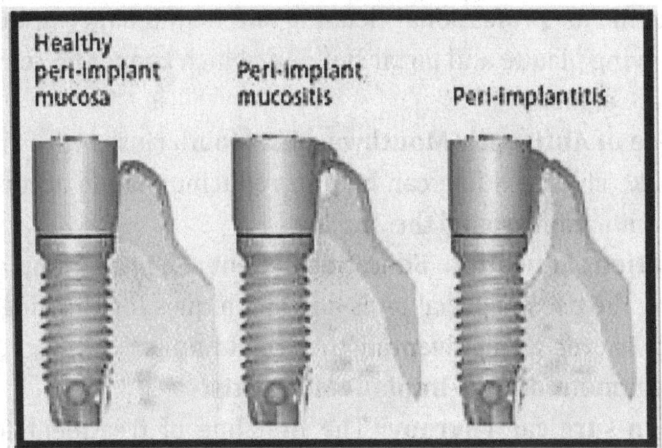

Peri-implant diseases are a significant concern in implant dentistry, affecting the long-term success of dental implants. These diseases are classified into two major categories:

1. **Peri-implant Mucositis**: A reversible inflammatory condition that affects the soft tissue around the implant, without bone loss. It is akin to gingivitis in natural teeth and can be caused by poor oral hygiene, bacterial accumulation, or smoking. Symptoms include redness, swelling, bleeding on probing, and discomfort.

2. **Peri-implantitis**: A more severe condition that involves both soft tissue inflammation and progressive bone loss around the implant. It can occur when peri-implant mucositis is left untreated and can lead to implant failure if not addressed promptly. Risk

factors include poor oral hygiene, smoking, systemic diseases (like diabetes), and a history of periodontal disease.

Prevention Strategies:

- **Proper Oral Hygiene**: The cornerstone of preventing both peri-implant mucositis and peri-implantitis is maintaining excellent oral hygiene. Regular brushing, flossing, and the use of interdental brushes are essential to prevent plaque accumulation around the implant.

- **Regular Professional Maintenance**: Periodic visits to the dental clinic for professional cleaning and maintenance are essential for removing plaque and tartar buildup, which cannot be removed by home care alone.

- **Use of Antiseptic Mouthwashes**: Mouth rinses with antiseptic agents like chlorhexidine can help in reducing plaque accumulation and inflammation around the implant.

- **Patient Education**: Educating patients on proper implant care, including the use of special tools and techniques for cleaning around implants, is crucial in preventing these conditions.

Management of Peri-Implant Mucositis:

- **Non-surgical Therapy**: The first line of treatment for peri-implant mucositis involves non-surgical methods to remove bacterial biofilms. This may include scaling and root planing (implant surface cleaning) with ultrasonic or hand instruments. The goal is to remove plaque and calculus from the implant surface without damaging it.

- **Use of Antiseptic Agents**: Rinsing with antiseptic mouthwashes like chlorhexidine can help reduce inflammation and bacterial load in the affected area.

- **Improved Home Care**: Ensuring the patient improves their home care regimen is essential. Dental professionals may recommend specific oral care tools, such as interdental brushes or water flossers, to clean around implants effectively.

Management of Peri-Implantitis:

- **Non-surgical Therapy**: If diagnosed early, peri-implantitis can often be treated without surgery. Non-surgical treatments include:

o **Mechanical Debridement**: Using instruments like titanium curettes or ultrasonic scalers to clean the implant surface.

o **Antibiotic Therapy**: Systemic or local antibiotics may be prescribed to control bacterial infection.

o **Laser Therapy**: Some studies suggest that laser treatment can help disinfect the implant surface and reduce inflammation, offering a non-invasive alternative to surgery.

- **Surgical Therapy**: In cases where non-surgical treatment fails or bone loss is severe, surgical intervention may be necessary. Surgical treatments may include:

o **Flap Surgery**: A procedure where the soft tissue around the implant is raised to access the affected area and clean the implant surface, followed by suturing to promote healing.

o **Bone Grafting**: If significant bone loss has occurred, bone grafting may be required to regenerate lost bone and restore the implant site.

o **Implant Removal**: In extreme cases of infection or implant failure, the implant may need to be removed to prevent further complications.

Role of Periodontists, Oral Surgeons, and Prosthodontists in Addressing Implant Complications

The management of peri-implant diseases requires a collaborative effort from periodontists, oral surgeons, and prosthodontists. Each specialist plays a vital role in preventing, diagnosing, and treating peri-implant diseases.

1. **Periodontists**:

Periodontists play a crucial role in maintaining the health and longevity of dental implants. Their expertise in the prevention, diagnosis, and treatment of periodontal diseases extends to managing conditions like peri-implant mucositis and peri-implantitis, which are inflammatory responses affecting peri-implant tissues. Here's a detailed elaboration:

1. Role in Assessing Peri-Implant Health

- **Evaluation of Periodontal and Peri-Implant Tissues:**

Periodontists conduct comprehensive examinations to assess the health of the gums and supporting bone around both natural teeth and implants.

- o **Key Diagnostic Tools:**
- Probing to measure pocket depths and identify inflammation or attachment loss.
- Radiographic analysis to detect bone loss or peri-implant radiolucencies.
- Microbiological testing to identify pathogens causing infection.
- o **Purpose:**

Early detection of peri-implant mucositis (reversible inflammation of soft tissue) to prevent progression to peri-implantitis (inflammatory bone loss).

2. Management of Peri-Implant Mucositis and Peri-Implantitis

- **Non-Surgical Interventions for Peri-Implant Mucositis:**
- o Scaling and root planing to remove plaque and biofilm from implant surfaces.
- o Use of adjunctive therapies such as antimicrobial mouth rinses (e.g., chlorhexidine) or localized antibiotics.
- o Laser-assisted therapy to target and reduce inflammation.
- **Advanced Management for Peri-Implantitis:**
- o When peri-implantitis has caused significant bone loss, surgical intervention may be required:
- **Flap Surgery:**
- A surgical procedure where the gum tissue is temporarily lifted to gain access to the implant surface and surrounding bone.
- Purpose: Thorough decontamination of the implant surface and removal of infected tissue.
- **Bone Regeneration Procedures:**
- Techniques such as guided bone regeneration (GBR) using membranes and grafts to restore lost bone.
- Purpose: Reinstate structural support for the implant and stabilize the surrounding bone.

3. Maintenance Therapy

- **Long-Term Implant Care:** Periodontists develop tailored maintenance protocols to ensure the health of peri-implant tissues post-treatment.
  o Regular cleaning and monitoring of implants to prevent biofilm accumulation.
  o Educating patients on optimal oral hygiene practices, including the use of specialized brushes and floss for implants.
  o Periodic professional cleanings to maintain the longevity of implants and surrounding tissues.

4. Additional Surgical Expertise
- In addition to managing infections, periodontists are skilled in other procedures critical to implant success, including:
  o **Soft Tissue Grafting:**
    ▪ Improves the quantity and quality of keratinized tissue around implants, reducing the risk of soft tissue recession.
  o **Ridge Augmentation:**
    ▪ Restores bone volume to support implant placement in cases of severe bone loss.

2. **Oral Surgeons**:
Oral surgeons play a vital role in managing the surgical complexities associated with dental implantology. Their expertise is essential in addressing advanced challenges and complications, ensuring the implant site's health and the success of the implant. Here's a detailed elaboration of their responsibilities:

1. Advanced Surgical Interventions

Bone Grafting
- **Purpose:**
Restores bone volume in areas with significant resorption or insufficient bone density, ensuring a stable foundation for implant placement.
- **Techniques:**
  o Autogenous bone grafts (from the patient's body).
  o Allografts, xenografts, or synthetic materials (alloplasts) as alternatives.

o   Ridge splitting or expansion to widen the alveolar ridge.

- **Role of the Surgeon:** Oral surgeons assess the defect, plan the grafting procedure, and perform precise placement of graft material to optimize bone regeneration.

Sinus Lifts

- **Purpose:**

Enhances bone height in the posterior maxilla by lifting the sinus membrane and placing graft material beneath it. This is crucial for implant placement in areas with reduced vertical bone.

- **Role of the Surgeon:** Oral surgeons ensure safe manipulation of the sinus membrane, avoiding complications such as membrane perforation or sinus infection.

Implant Removal

- **Purpose:**

Necessary when implants fail due to severe peri-implantitis, fractures, or lack of osseointegration.

- **Role of the Surgeon:**

o   Perform atraumatic removal of the failed implant to minimize damage to surrounding bone.

o   Prepare the site for future implant placement using grafting or regenerative techniques.

2. Managing Complications

Implant Fractures

- **Nature of the Complication:** Implants may fracture due to excessive occlusal forces, design flaws, or manufacturing defects.

- **Role of the Surgeon:**

o   Assess the extent of the fracture and determine whether removal or repair is feasible.

o   If removal is required, the surgeon carefully extracts the fractured implant and prepares the site for rehabilitation.

Severe Bone Loss

- **Nature of the Complication:** Severe bone loss around an implant can result from peri-implantitis, trauma, or systemic conditions affecting bone metabolism.

- **Role of the Surgeon:**
o Perform surgical debridement to remove infected tissue and contaminated implant surfaces.
o Utilize advanced bone regeneration techniques to restore lost bone and improve implant site health.

3. Collaborative Approach

Oral surgeons often work closely with periodontists, prosthodontists, and restorative dentists to:
- Develop comprehensive treatment plans addressing both functional and aesthetic goals.
- Coordinate timing and procedures for optimal outcomes, such as performing grafting before implant placement or managing soft tissue concerns post-operatively.

4. Ensuring Long-Term Success

- Oral surgeons contribute to implant success by addressing challenges with precision and care:
o Stabilizing implants in challenging cases such as compromised bone conditions or anatomical complexities.
o Utilizing advanced imaging (CBCT) for precise planning and execution.
o Managing post-operative complications to ensure rapid healing and site integrity.

3. **Prosthodontists**:

Prosthodontists play a pivotal role in the final stages of dental implant treatment, focusing on the design, fabrication, and placement of the prosthetic restoration. Their expertise ensures the implant restoration is both functional and esthetically pleasing while minimizing stress on surrounding tissues. Here is a detailed explanation of their responsibilities:

1. Design and Placement of Prosthetic Restorations

Designing the Restoration:
- **Individualized Treatment Planning:** Prosthodontists consider factors like occlusion, esthetics, and patient-specific anatomical conditions when designing the prosthesis.

o **Occlusion:** Ensures proper bite alignment to avoid overloading the implant.

o **Esthetics:** Focuses on achieving a natural appearance, particularly for restorations in the anterior region.

o **Material Selection:** Chooses appropriate materials such as zirconia, porcelain, or metal-based restorations based on durability and esthetic requirements.

Placement of the Prosthesis:

• **Precision Fit:** Ensures that the prosthetic crown, bridge, or denture fits accurately onto the implant abutment to avoid undue stress.

o Poorly fitting restorations can lead to micromovements, resulting in inflammation or peri-implant bone loss.

• **Alignment and Load Distribution:**

o Proper alignment of the restoration prevents excessive forces on the implant or surrounding bone, reducing the risk of complications like screw loosening or implant failure.

2. Communication with Periodontists

Collaborative Treatment Planning:

• **Pre-Restoration Assessment:** Periodontists evaluate peri-implant tissue health and bone stability before prosthesis placement. Prosthodontists use this information to guide the design and placement process.

• **Shared Goals:**

o Periodontists ensure the implant is surrounded by healthy tissues.

o Prosthodontists focus on ensuring the restoration maintains these tissues by avoiding improper occlusion or poor fit.

Prevention of Peri-Implant Diseases:

• **Role of Occlusion:**

o Misaligned prosthetic restorations can create excessive stress on the implant, leading to peri-implantitis.

o Prosthodontists work with periodontists to ensure balanced occlusion that avoids overloading the implant.

- **Soft Tissue Management:**
o Prosthodontists ensure that restorations allow for adequate hygiene access, minimizing the risk of biofilm accumulation and soft tissue inflammation.

3. Supporting Esthetic and Functional Outcomes

Esthetic Considerations:

- **Anterior Restorations:**
o Focus on matching the natural tooth shade, shape, and contour to achieve a seamless appearance.
- **Gingival Integration:**
o Works with periodontists to ensure harmonious integration of the prosthesis with the surrounding soft tissues for a natural gumline.

Functional Considerations:

- **Bite Force Distribution:**
o Ensures the prosthesis distributes forces evenly across the implant and adjacent teeth, reducing stress on any one component.
- **Speech and Comfort:**
o Adjustments are made to ensure the restoration does not impair speech or cause discomfort during chewing.

---

4. Long-Term Maintenance and Monitoring

- **Regular Follow-Ups:** Prosthodontists play an ongoing role in monitoring the health of the prosthesis and the underlying implant.
- **Prosthesis Repairs or Adjustments:**
o Replacing worn crowns or bridges.
o Adjusting occlusion to accommodate changes in the patient's bite over time.

Surgical and Non-Surgical Treatments for Peri-Implant Diseases

1. **Non-surgical Treatments:**
o **Implant Surface Cleaning:** Mechanical debridement with instruments specifically designed for use on titanium surfaces, such as ultrasonic scalers or plastic curettes, helps to remove bacterial

biofilm from the implant surface without causing damage.

o **Antimicrobial Therapy**: The use of local and systemic antibiotics (such as tetracycline or metronidazole) can help control infection and inflammation around the implant.

o **Laser Therapy**: Lasers have been shown to effectively decontaminate the implant surface and reduce bacterial load in peri-implantitis cases. The use of diode or erbium lasers has shown promising results in treating peri-implant diseases.

Surgical Treatments:

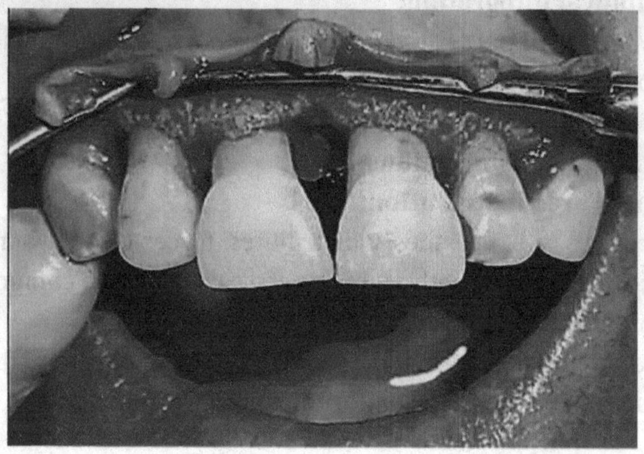

Flap Surgery: This procedure allows for direct access to the implant surface to clean the affected area. Flap surgery also enables the removal of granulation tissue and infected bone, followed by bone grafting if necessary.

o **Bone Grafting**: If peri-implantitis has led to significant bone loss, bone grafting can restore the lost bone and improve the stability of the implant. Various grafting materials (autografts, allografts, xenografts) can be used depending on the case.

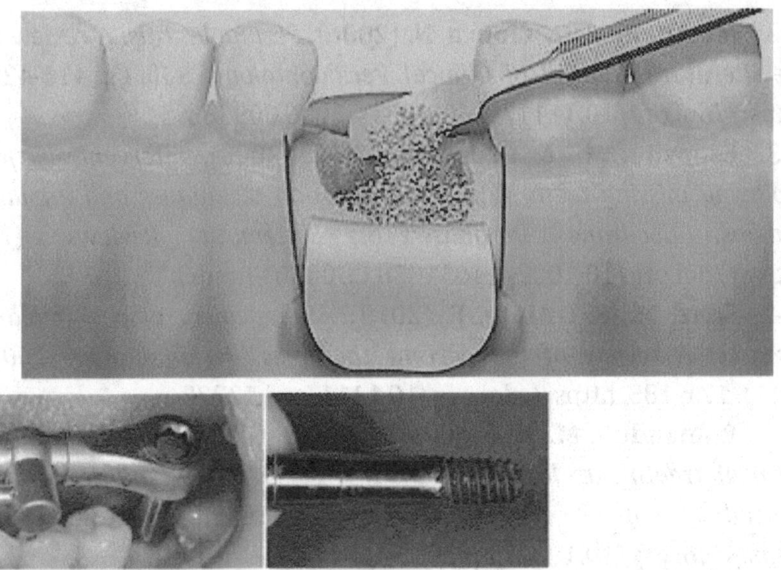

Resection and Implant Removal: In severe cases where the implant is no longer salvageable, removal of the implant may be necessary, followed by reestablishment of bone and tissue health before a new implant is placed.

Conclusion

Peri-implant diseases, particularly peri-implant mucositis and peri-implantitis, are significant challenges in implant dentistry. Early detection, prevention, and appropriate treatment are crucial to preserving implant function and longevity. An interdisciplinary approach involving periodontists, oral surgeons, and prosthodontists ensures comprehensive care that addresses both the soft and hard tissue issues surrounding the implant. By working together, these specialists can provide effective solutions, from non-surgical treatments to complex surgical interventions, ultimately ensuring successful and cost-effective implant therapy.

References:

1. **Lang, N. P., & Berglundh, T.** (2011). *Periimplant diseases: Changing the paradigm. Journal of Clinical Periodontology*, 38(Suppl 11), 1-4. https://doi.org/10.1111/j.1600-051X.2010.01694.x

2. **Mombelli, A., & Cionca, N.** (2006). *Periimplantitis: A review of the literature. Journal of Clinical Periodontology*, 33(11), 416-428. https://doi.org/10.1111/j.1600-051X.2006.00958.x

3. **Esposito, M., & Grusovin, M. G.** (2008). *Interventions for replacing missing teeth: Bone augmentation techniques and implant systems. Cochrane Database of Systematic Reviews*, (2). https://doi.org/10.1002/14651858.CD003041.pub3

4. **Sanz, M., & D'Aiuto, F.** (2019). *Management of peri-implant diseases: A review of the current therapies. Periodontology 2000*, 79(1), 171-185. https://doi.org/10.1111/prd.12278

5. **Romandini, M., & Tatakis, D. N.** (2015). *Effectiveness of non-surgical treatments for peri-implant diseases: A systematic review. Journal of Periodontology*, 86(11), 1340-1350. https://doi.org/10.1902/jop.2015.150170

Chapter 8

Restorative and Periodontal Interface in Implant Success

Dr. Prateek Mishra

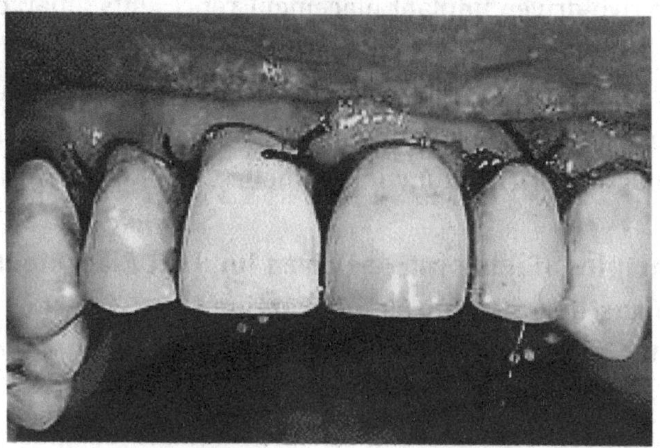

Restorative-driven implant placement has become a standard approach in implant dentistry, ensuring that the final prosthesis aligns with both functional and aesthetic goals. The collaboration between restorative and periodontal specialists plays a pivotal role in achieving implant success, especially when aligning restorative goals with the health of the periodontal tissues.

Restorative-Driven Implant Placement: Aligning Restorative Goals with Periodontal Health

Restorative-driven implant placement emphasizes the importance of planning implant positions based on the final prosthetic design rather than merely focusing on the implant's structural placement. This method considers the future restoration's position, size, and shape, ensuring that the implant is optimally positioned for both function and aesthetics. Importantly, this approach requires collaboration between the restorative dentist, periodontist, and implant surgeon to assess the surrounding tissues and the available bone structure. In India, the growing accessibility of advanced imaging techniques like CBCT (Cone Beam Computed Tomography) has facilitated more accurate and predictable restorative-driven implant planning. By planning restorations from the start, practitioners can better ensure the health of the peri-implant tissues, leading to better long-term outcomes.

Restorative-driven implant placement represents a paradigm shift in dental implantology, emphasizing the planning of implant placement based on the anticipated prosthetic restoration rather than focusing solely on anatomical or structural considerations. This methodology prioritizes function, esthetics, and long-term success.

1. Principles of Restorative-Driven Implant Placement
Final Prosthetic Design as the Starting Point
- **Functionality:** The implant is placed to support the optimal bite (occlusion) and ensure efficient chewing dynamics.
- **Esthetics:** The position of the implant ensures the final restoration blends seamlessly with the surrounding dentition and soft tissue. This is particularly critical for anterior teeth, where even minor deviations can compromise appearance.
- **Prosthetic Stability:** Proper planning prevents complications like misaligned restorations, excessive stress on implants, or the need for prosthetic adjustments.

Key Considerations:
- **Positioning:** The angle and depth of implant placement are determined by the restoration's shape and alignment with adjacent teeth.
- **Emergence Profile:** The implant's placement must allow the crown to emerge naturally from the gum line, mimicking the appearance of natural teeth.
- **Soft Tissue and Bone Support:** Ensures adequate bone and gingival support to maintain the health of peri-implant tissues.

2. Collaborative Planning and Multidisciplinary Approach

Restorative-driven implant placement requires close collaboration between the following specialists:

- **Restorative Dentist:** Designs the final prosthetic restoration and communicates its requirements to the surgical team.
- **Periodontist:** Evaluates the health of peri-implant tissues and performs soft and hard tissue augmentation if needed to support the planned restoration.
- **Oral Surgeon/Implantologist:** Places the implant in a precise position guided by the restorative plan, ensuring optimal integration with the surrounding structures.

Steps in Collaborative Planning:

1. **Initial Assessment:**
   - Collecting patient history, imaging, and impressions to design a preliminary prosthetic plan.
2. **Bone and Soft Tissue Evaluation:**
   - Using advanced imaging techniques to assess bone density, height, and soft tissue volume.
3. **Guided Implant Placement:**
   - Utilizing surgical guides or navigation systems to place implants according to the restorative blueprint.

3. Role of CBCT in Restorative-Driven Planning

In India, the increasing availability of advanced imaging techniques like CBCT (Cone Beam Computed Tomography) has revolutionized restorative-driven implant planning:

- **Enhanced Precision:** CBCT provides 3D visualization of bone structure, surrounding tissues, and vital anatomical landmarks (e.g., sinuses, nerves).
- **Virtual Planning:** Digital workflows allow for the simulation of implant placement relative to the final prosthetic design.
- **Custom Surgical Guides:** CBCT data is used to fabricate guides that ensure implants are placed in precise positions according

to the prosthetic plan.

Benefits in Clinical Practice:

- **Reduced Errors:** Prevents improper placement that could compromise esthetics or function.
- **Predictable Outcomes:** Increases the likelihood of long-term implant success by aligning surgical and restorative goals.
- **Time Efficiency:** Minimizes the need for post-surgical adjustments or revisions.

---

4. Advantages of Restorative-Driven Implant Placement

1. **Optimal Esthetic Outcomes:**
   - Ensures natural-looking restorations that align with the patient's smile and facial symmetry.
2. **Improved Functionality:**
   - Restorations fit comfortably and perform effectively in daily activities.
3. **Healthier Peri-Implant Tissues:**
   - Reduces the risk of peri-implant diseases by promoting proper bone integration and minimizing stress on soft tissues.
4. **Patient Satisfaction:**
   - Aesthetic and functional results lead to higher satisfaction and confidence.
5. **Cost-Effectiveness:**
   - Avoids additional procedures for correction, saving time and resources.

Managing Soft Tissue Around Restorative Crowns for Optimal Gingival Aesthetics

The soft tissue around dental implants plays a crucial role in the overall appearance of the restoration. Gingival aesthetics, particularly the contour, color, and texture of the gum tissue around the crown, significantly impact the final outcome of the implant treatment. Managing soft tissue is a key element for achieving a natural look, and the periodontist's role in shaping the peri-implant tissues is crucial. Techniques such as soft tissue grafting, contouring, and the use of custom healing abutments can aid in achieving optimal soft tissue support for the restorative crown. Furthermore, the careful consideration of the crown's contour can help manage the surrounding soft tissue, preventing complications such as mucosal recession or overgrowth.

In India, where there is a growing emphasis on aesthetics, especially in urban populations, achieving high-quality gingival aesthetics through collaborative treatment planning is increasingly valued. This is further facilitated by the availability of advanced prosthetic materials and techniques that promote a more seamless integration of the implant crown with the surrounding gingival tissue.

Soft tissue health and aesthetics play a vital role in the success and appearance of dental implants. The soft tissue around implants not only impacts the visual appeal of the restoration but also contributes to its functional and biological stability.

1. Importance of Gingival Aesthetics

The gingival tissues around the implant crown significantly influence the treatment's final outcome. Key factors include:

- **Contour:**

The natural scalloping of the gum line ensures a harmonious transition between the restoration and the adjacent teeth.

- **Color:**

Healthy gum tissue matches the color of the surrounding gingiva, avoiding discoloration or visible margins.

- **Texture:**

A natural stippled appearance adds to the restoration's realism.

Achieving these qualities enhances patient satisfaction, especially in anterior restorations where esthetics are paramount.

2. Techniques for Soft Tissue Management

Periodontists and implantologists employ various techniques to optimize soft tissue support:

a. Soft Tissue Grafting:
- **Purpose:**

Improves tissue volume and quality around implants.
- **Types:**
- o **Connective Tissue Grafts:** Commonly used to thicken tissues and prevent recession.
- o **Free Gingival Grafts:** Enhance keratinized tissue width, essential for peri-implant health.

b. Tissue Contouring:
- Reshaping the gum tissue around the implant crown to mimic natural tooth contours and create an esthetically pleasing outcome.

c. Custom Healing Abutments:
- Abutments designed to mold the peri-implant tissue during the healing phase, ensuring a natural emergence profile for the prosthesis.

d. Proper Crown Design:
- The shape and emergence profile of the implant crown influence the positioning and health of the surrounding soft tissue. A well-contoured crown prevents:
- o **Mucosal Recession:** Exposure of the implant or crown margins.
- o **Overgrowth:** Excessive tissue covering the crown.

---

3. Collaboration for Enhanced Aesthetic Outcomes
Achieving optimal soft tissue aesthetics requires a multidisciplinary approach:
- **Periodontist:** Shapes and maintains the peri-implant tissue health through surgical and non-surgical methods.
- **Prosthodontist:** Designs restorations that complement soft tissue contours and appearance.
- **Implant Surgeon:** Ensures proper implant positioning to support soft tissue esthetics.

---

4. Advanced Prosthetic Materials and Techniques

In India, the emphasis on esthetics is growing, particularly in urban areas where patients prioritize natural-looking restorations. This trend has been supported by advancements in:

Prosthetic Materials:

- Zirconia-based restorations: Offer superior esthetics and compatibility with soft tissues.
- Pink porcelain: Mimics gingival tissue in cases where soft tissue deficiencies exist.

Digital Techniques:

- **CAD/CAM technology:** Enables precise customization of restorations to match the gingival profile.
- **Digital Smile Design (DSD):** Helps visualize and plan soft tissue and prosthetic outcomes.

5. Challenges and Considerations

- **Mucosal Recession:** Can occur if soft tissues are not adequately managed or if the implant placement is suboptimal.
- **Peri-Implant Inflammation:** Poor tissue management or improper prosthetic design can lead to soft tissue irritation.
- **Patient Factors:** Smoking, oral hygiene practices, and systemic conditions (e.g., diabetes) may influence soft tissue health.

Interdisciplinary Focus on Prosthetic Margins and Their Impact on Peri-Implant Tissue

The prosthetic margins, the edge of the restoration where it meets the gingiva, are critical in determining the success of the implant restoration, particularly concerning the health of the peri-implant tissues. The prosthodontist's role in selecting the correct margin design can help reduce the likelihood of inflammation, plaque accumulation, and soft tissue recession. A poorly designed margin can lead to the development of peri-implant mucositis or peri-implantitis. Therefore, collaboration with the periodontist is necessary to ensure that the margin design respects the biological width and soft tissue contour, promoting optimal health around the implant site.

Moreover, careful attention to the transition between the crown and the soft tissue helps maintain a proper balance between the prosthetic and periodontal health. A well-designed margin should facilitate cleaning by the patient and avoid trauma to the surrounding tissue during both the prosthetic placement and daily oral hygiene routines.

Crown-to-Soft Tissue Transition: Balancing Prosthetic and Periodontal Health

The transition zone between the implant crown and the soft tissue is a critical factor in ensuring both functional and esthetic success in implant dentistry. This delicate interface demands meticulous planning and execution to maintain prosthetic stability and periodontal health while allowing for effective patient maintenance.

Key Considerations for a Successful Transition

1. **Margin Design and Placement:**

o **Subgingival Margins:** Typically used for esthetics in anterior regions, but must be placed cautiously to avoid excessive depth that may compromise cleaning or irritate the peri-implant tissues.

o **Equigingival/Supragingival Margins:** Preferred in posterior regions to facilitate hygiene and reduce inflammation risks.

2. **Smooth and Accessible Margins:**

o Well-polished margins minimize plaque retention and reduce the risk of peri-implant diseases.

o Margins should transition seamlessly into the soft tissue, ensuring no overhangs that could cause irritation or impede cleaning.

Facilitating Effective Cleaning and Maintenance

A well-designed transition should:

- **Allow Easy Access for Oral Hygiene:**

o Encourage patient compliance with daily cleaning using tools like interdental brushes or water flossers.

o Avoid areas where food and plaque could accumulate.

- **Minimize Trauma:**
  o Smooth contours prevent tissue irritation during routine cleaning or mastication.
  o Proper emergence profiles help distribute forces evenly on the soft tissues.

Protecting the Surrounding Tissue

1. **During Prosthetic Placement:**
   o Careful handling of the peri-implant tissues during crown placement minimizes trauma and inflammation.
   o Use of non-irritating materials like zirconia or titanium abutments ensures biocompatibility.
2. **Post-Placement Maintenance:**
   o Educate patients on maintaining the crown-tissue interface using appropriate hygiene tools.
   o Schedule regular follow-ups for professional cleaning and monitoring of tissue health.

Balancing Esthetics and Function

- **Esthetics:**
  o A smooth transition maintains a natural-looking gumline and prevents mucosal recession.
  o Custom abutments and proper crown contouring help integrate the prosthetic seamlessly with surrounding tissues.
- **Function:**
  o The transition zone must withstand masticatory forces without causing tissue irritation or inflammation.
  o Proper occlusal design ensures forces are distributed evenly, reducing strain on the implant and adjacent tissues.

Economic Considerations in Restorative and Periodontal Integration

In India, economic considerations are crucial when integrating restorative and periodontal care. While the interdisciplinary approach may seem costly at first glance, it leads to greater long-term cost-efficiency by preventing complications and ensuring the long-term success of the implant. For example, treating peri-implant diseases at an early stage and paying attention to the management of soft tissues can reduce the need for expensive corrective procedures later on.

By strategically planning the restorative and periodontal aspects of implant therapy from the beginning, dental practitioners can reduce the need for corrective treatments and ensure that the patient's investment in implant dentistry yields lasting results. Additionally, the integration of cost-effective materials and techniques, such as pre-fabricated abutments and minimally invasive soft tissue management procedures, can help provide affordable care without compromising quality.

Table 1: Economic Comparison of Restorative and Periodontal Integration Approaches in Implant Dentistry

Procedure	Traditional Approach Cost (INR)	Restorative-Driven Implant Placement with Periodontal Integration Cost (INR)	Potential Savings
Implant Placement	25,000 - 40,000	30,000 - 45,000	10%
Soft Tissue Management (Grafting, Contouring)	5,000 - 10,000	7,000 - 15,000	5%
Prosthetic Crown (Standard)	15,000 - 30,000	18,000 - 35,000	5%
Peri-implant Disease Treatment	10,000 - 20,000	5,000 - 15,000 (preventative)	20%
Total Treatment Cost	55,000 - 100,000	60,000 - 95,000	10-20%

Note: Costs are approximate and vary by region, clinic, and treatment complexity. Restorative-driven approaches may initially have higher costs due to the need for more detailed planning and collaboration, but the overall savings from reduced complications can make these approaches more cost-effective in the long term.

References:

1. **Jaffin, R. A., & Berman, C. L.** (1991). *The excessive loss of implants in patients with a history of periodontal disease. Journal of Periodontology*, 62(2), 77-83.

2. **Piñeiro, A., & González, I.** (2014). *Soft tissue management around dental implants: Biological principles and clinical considerations. Journal of Prosthetic Dentistry*, 112(5), 1009-1016.

3. **Albrektsson, T., & Zarb, G.** (1993). *Osseointegration: A paradigm shift in implant dentistry. Journal of Prosthetic Dentistry*, 70(1), 7-12.

4. **Sanz, M., & Cecchinato, D.** (2016). *Periodontal surgery for dental implants: A collaborative approach with restorative and prosthodontic specialists. Periodontology 2000*, 72(1), 90-99.

5. **Esposito, M., & Grusovin, M. G.** (2010). *Interventions for replacing missing teeth: Bone augmentation techniques and implant systems. Cochrane Database of Systematic Reviews*, (2). https://doi.org/10.1002/14651858.CD003041.pub3

Chapter 9

Immediate implant placement

Dr. Rahul Anand Razdan

The procedure where an implant is placed directly after tooth extraction, is a widely utilized technique in modern implant dentistry. This method offers several advantages, such as reduced treatment time, preservation of bone and soft tissues, and enhanced patient comfort. However, immediate implant placement requires a high level of coordination between multiple dental disciplines, including surgery, periodontics, and prosthodontics, to ensure a successful outcome.

Immediate Implant Placement: A Multidisciplinary Approach to Modern Implant Dentistry

Immediate implant placement, where the dental implant is placed immediately following tooth extraction, has revolutionized implantology by offering faster and more efficient treatment pathways. This technique comes with numerous benefits but requires meticulous planning and collaboration among dental disciplines to ensure long-term success.

Advantages of Immediate Implant Placement

1. Reduced Treatment Time:

o **Eliminates the need for a prolonged healing phase after tooth extraction, shortening the overall treatment duration.**

o **Enhances patient satisfaction by providing quicker restoration of function and esthetics.**

2. Preservation of Hard and Soft Tissues:

o **Immediate placement minimizes alveolar bone resorption, maintaining the natural ridge contour.**

o Helps preserve the surrounding gingival architecture, enhancing the esthetic outcome.

3. Improved Patient Comfort:

o Fewer surgical interventions reduce postoperative discomfort and anxiety.

o A single surgical event decreases overall recovery time.

Challenges and Considerations

1. Socket Morphology:

o The extraction socket's dimensions and the quality of surrounding bone must be adequate for primary implant stability.

o Additional bone grafting may be required if bone defects are present.

2. Primary Stability:

o Achieving sufficient initial implant stability is crucial for osseointegration. This often involves engaging the apical or lateral native bone.

3. Soft Tissue Management:

o Careful handling of gingival tissues is necessary to preserve the natural esthetics and prevent recession.

o Soft tissue grafts may be needed to optimize the peri-implant tissue contours.

4. Risk of Infection:

o A thorough debridement of the socket is essential to remove infected or necrotic tissue and minimize contamination risks.

Multidisciplinary Collaboration

1. Surgical Expertise:

o Oral surgeons or periodontists assess and prepare the extraction site, ensuring optimal bone quality and implant placement.

o Techniques like flapless surgery can be employed to

minimize soft tissue trauma.

2. Periodontal Management:

o **Periodontists play a role in assessing and maintaining the health of peri-implant tissues.**

o **They perform bone augmentation procedures when necessary and address any soft tissue deficiencies.**

3. Prosthodontic Input:

o **Prosthodontists ensure that the implant placement aligns with the future prosthetic design for optimal function and esthetics.**

o **Immediate temporary restorations may be provided to support soft tissue shaping during healing.**

Indications for Immediate Implant Placement and the Need for Interdisciplinary Planning

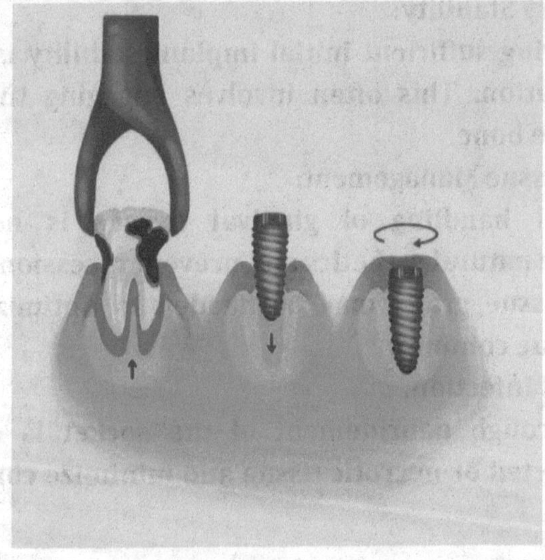

Immediate implant placement is typically indicated in cases where the extracted tooth is severely damaged or decayed but the surrounding bone and soft tissue are still healthy. Ideal candidates for this procedure include patients with sufficient bone volume, absence of infection, and favorable root morphology. The patient's overall health and the ability to maintain oral hygiene also play critical roles in determining whether immediate implant placement is appropriate.

The need for interdisciplinary planning is crucial when performing immediate implant placements. Coordination between the oral surgeon, periodontist, and prosthodontist ensures that the surgical procedure is planned meticulously and that the final restoration aligns with both functional and aesthetic goals. A thorough evaluation of the extraction site is essential to assess factors like bone volume, tissue health, and the position of adjacent teeth. In cases where immediate restoration is planned, the prosthodontist's input regarding the desired esthetic outcome, occlusal considerations, and material selection is key to achieving a satisfactory result.

In India, where advancements in dental technology and implant systems have become more accessible, the success of immediate implant placement has greatly improved. Innovations such as digital radiography and 3D imaging assist in accurately assessing the extraction site and planning for immediate implant placement, leading to higher success rates and predictable outcomes.

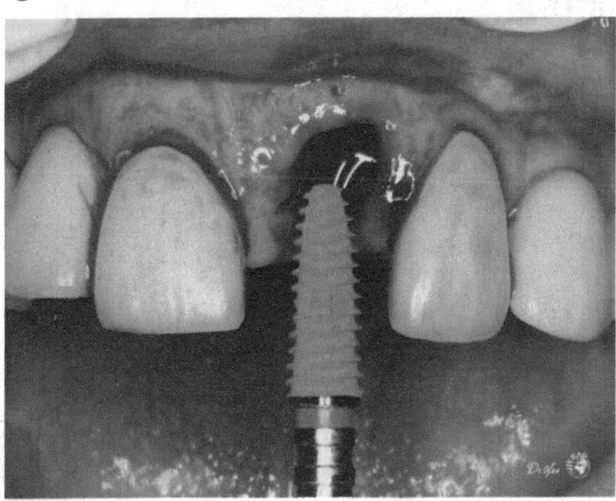

Periodontal and Surgical Considerations for Extraction and Implant Placement in One Visit

Immediate implant placement has numerous benefits, but it

requires careful periodontal and surgical planning to avoid complications. After tooth extraction, it is crucial to assess the health and volume of the surrounding periodontal tissues, including the alveolar bone, the gingiva, and the connective tissues. The surgeon must ensure that there is adequate bone support for the implant and that the extraction site is free of infection.

The surgical procedure for immediate implant placement often involves the use of guided bone regeneration (GBR) techniques or socket preservation procedures to maintain the alveolar bone's integrity. If there is insufficient bone volume, the periodontist and surgeon may decide to augment the site using bone grafts or soft tissue grafts to ensure the long-term stability of the implant.

The success of the immediate implant placement is influenced by how well the periodontal tissues are managed during the extraction and implant placement procedure. Proper flap design and the careful handling of soft tissue around the implant are essential to achieving favorable results. The periodontist plays a significant role in optimizing the health of the periodontal tissues before, during, and after the surgery.

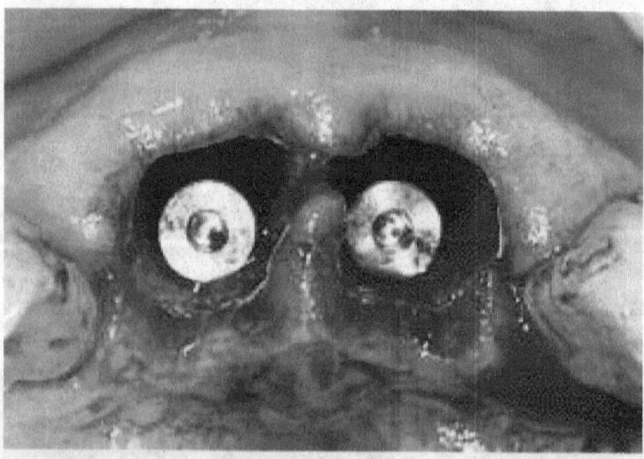

Prosthodontic Role in Designing Immediate Restorations that Respect Periodontal Health

The prosthodontist's role in immediate implant placement goes beyond designing the final restoration; it includes ensuring that the temporary restoration is properly designed to support the implant and the surrounding tissues. The immediate provisional restoration, placed on the implant shortly after surgery, serves as a scaffold to guide soft tissue healing and contour. The prosthodontist must design the restoration to mimic the natural contours of the adjacent teeth, ensuring it does not interfere with the healing of the surrounding gum tissue.

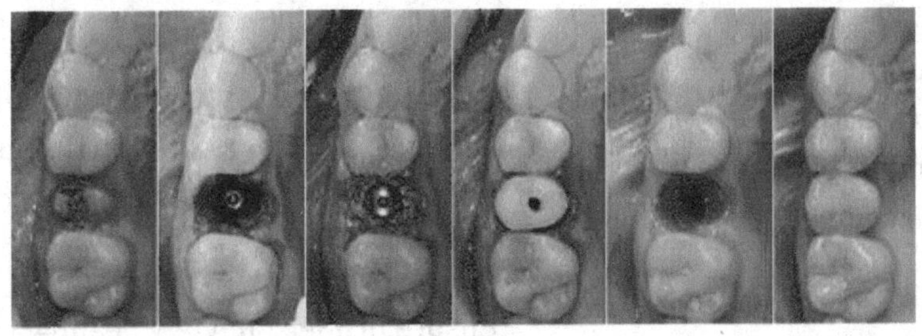

One of the key challenges of immediate restoration is balancing the need for aesthetic outcomes with the importance of preserving the health of the periodontal tissues. The immediate restoration must be designed to allow proper tissue healing and prevent tissue overgrowth or recession, which can affect the long-term success of the implant. Over-contouring or under-contouring of the restoration can lead to issues such as peri-implantitis or soft tissue recession. Therefore, the prosthodontist must work closely with the periodontist to ensure that the implant placement and restoration do not compromise the health of the surrounding tissues.

Additionally, the prosthodontist should be mindful of the materials used in the restoration, as the choice of material can influence both the esthetic outcome and the longevity of the implant. Materials such as zirconia or titanium are commonly used for temporary restorations due to their durability and aesthetic properties.

Table 1: Benefits of Immediate Implant Placement with Interdisciplinary Collaboration

Step in Treatment Process	Role of Surgeon	Role of Periodontist	Role of Prosthodontist
Pre-Surgical Evaluation	Assess bone and soft tissue health	Evaluate periodontal status, plan for bone grafts if needed	Ensure alignment with esthetic and functional goals
Tooth Extraction and Implant Placement	Extract tooth and place implant	Manage soft tissues, control bleeding, maintain tissue health	Assist in provisional restoration design and occlusion
Post-Surgical Care	Monitor implant stability, check for infection	Ensure proper healing of tissues, monitor for complications	Review healing and esthetics of provisional restoration
Final Restoration	Ensure implant integration	Evaluate soft tissue response and support	Design final restoration and ensure functional and esthetic outcome

Economic Considerations in Immediate Implant Placement

Immediate implant placement is often seen as an expensive procedure due to the complexity of the treatment and the need for multiple specialties to collaborate. However, when considering the long-term benefits, immediate implants can be more cost-effective compared to traditional implant protocols, which may require multiple visits and procedures such as bone grafting, healing periods, and additional surgeries. In India, the growing demand for faster and more cost-effective dental treatments has increased the popularity of immediate implants, particularly among patients who prefer quick recovery times and reduced treatment duration.

Cost-effective strategies for implementing immediate implants include utilizing advanced implant systems that allow for single-stage surgery, reducing the need for multiple visits. Furthermore, improvements in surgical techniques and materials, including the use of digital planning, have made immediate implant placement more affordable for patients.

Table 2: Economic Comparison of Immediate Implant Placement vs. Traditional Implant Protocol

Procedure	Traditional Protocol Cost (INR)	Immediate Implant Placement Cost (INR)	Potential Savings
Initial Consultation and Diagnosis	2,000 - 5,000	2,500 - 5,000	-
Tooth Extraction and Bone Grafting	8,000 - 15,000	10,000 - 18,000	10-15%
Implant Placement (Single Stage)	25,000 - 40,000	30,000 - 45,000	5-10%
Provisional Restoration	5,000 - 8,000	6,000 - 10,000	10%
Final Restoration	15,000 - 25,000	18,000 - 30,000	5-10%
Total Cost	55,000 - 95,000	60,000 - 95,000	5-20%

Note: Costs are approximate and vary by region, clinic, and treatment complexity. Immediate implants can reduce the overall treatment timeline, but may initially have higher costs due to the immediate provisional restoration and intensive surgical planning.

References:

1. **Chen, S. T., & Buser, D.** (2009). *Implant placement in the esthetic zone: A literature review on surgical and restorative considerations. International Journal of Oral & Maxillofacial Implants,* 24(6), 186-202.

2. **Curi, M. M., & Oliveira, G. R.** (2017). *Immediate implantation and restoration: Concepts and clinical perspectives. Brazilian Dental Journal,* 28(2), 160-165. https://doi.org/10.1590/0103-6440201700897

3. **Simion, M., & Mazzocco, M.** (2010). *Immediate implant placement after tooth extraction: A review of the current evidence and clinical recommendations. Journal of Oral Implantology,* 36(2), 83-92. https://doi.org/10.1563/AAID-JOI-D-10-00017

4. **Oates, T. W., & Sanz, M.** (2016). *The role of the periodontist in immediate implant placement and restoration. Periodontology 2000,* 71(1), 58-73. https://doi.org/10.1111/prd.12107

5. **Esposito, M., & Grusovin, M. G.** (2010). *Interventions for replacing missing teeth: Bone augmentation techniques and implant systems. Cochrane Database of Systematic Reviews,* (2). https://doi.org/10.1002/14651858.CD003041.pub3

Chapter 10

Oral Surgery in Managing Complex Implant Cases

Dr. Rahul Anand Razdan

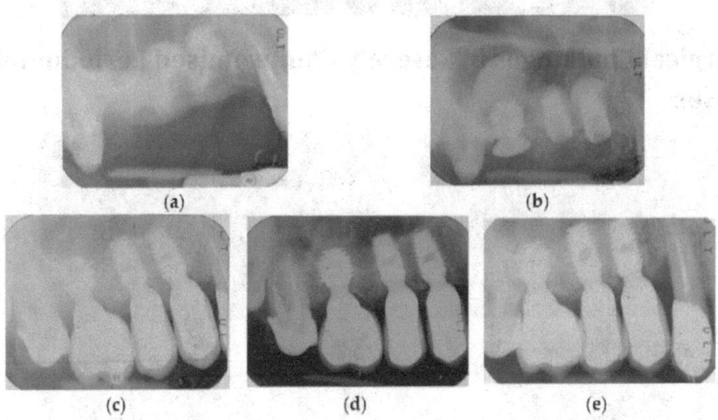

(a)   (b)
(c)   (d)   (e)

Managing complex implant cases often requires the combined expertise of oral surgeons, periodontists, and prosthodontists to ensure successful outcomes. These cases frequently involve patients with severe bone loss, compromised periodontal conditions, or other anatomical challenges that make traditional implant placement difficult. Oral surgery plays a pivotal role in overcoming these challenges by addressing structural issues, preparing the site for implant placement, and ensuring optimal conditions for long-term implant success.

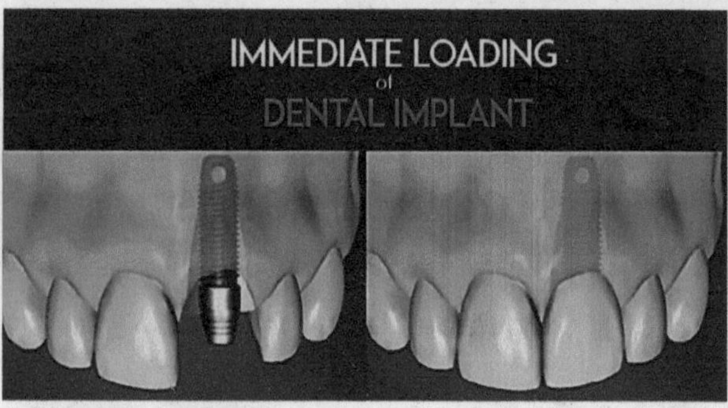

Surgical Challenges in Severely Compromised Periodontal Cases

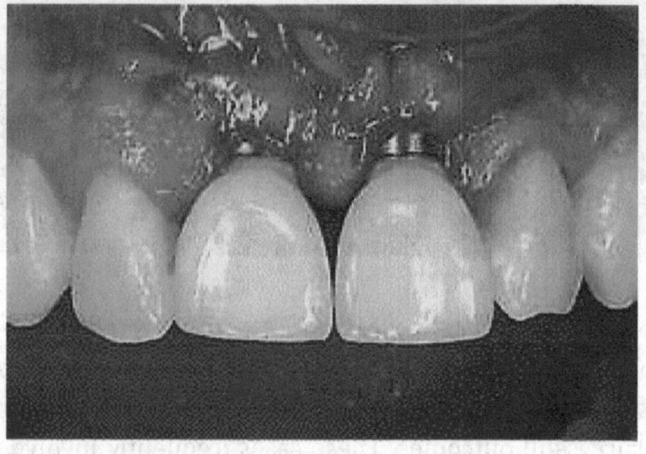

Severely compromised periodontal cases present several challenges for implant placement. Patients with advanced periodontitis or aggressive periodontal disease often experience significant bone resorption and soft tissue damage, which can complicate the process of placing implants. The lack of sufficient bone volume, especially in the upper and lower jaw areas, poses one of the biggest challenges, as it may be difficult to place an implant without proper support.

In these cases, careful evaluation and meticulous planning are critical. Oral surgeons must assess the level of bone resorption and determine whether bone grafting, guided bone regeneration (GBR), or sinus lift procedures are required. Surgical interventions in these cases often involve the use of autogenous bone grafts, allografts, or xenografts to restore bone volume. For patients with severe periodontal disease, addressing the underlying infection and restoring periodontal health is necessary before considering implant placement.

Implant Placement in Severely Compromised Periodontal Cases: Overcoming Challenges

Patients with advanced periodontal disease or aggressive periodontitis present significant challenges for implant placement due to extensive bone and soft tissue loss. Successfully restoring function and aesthetics in such cases requires a comprehensive, multidisciplinary approach.

Key Challenges in Periodontally Compromised Cases

1. **Severe Bone Resorption:**
o Advanced periodontitis often leads to significant bone loss, making it difficult to achieve primary stability for implants.
o Critical areas, such as the posterior maxilla (due to pneumatized sinuses) and mandible, are frequently affected.

2. **Soft Tissue Damage:**
o Gingival recession and compromised soft tissue health can impact the esthetic outcome and peri-implant tissue stability.

3. **Residual Periodontal Infections:**
o Active infection and inflammation need to be eradicated to ensure a healthy environment for implant osseointegration.

4. **Patient Systemic Conditions:**
o Severe periodontal disease is often associated with systemic conditions (e.g., diabetes), which can further compromise healing and implant success.

Approach to Implant Placement

1. **Comprehensive Evaluation and Planning:**
o Detailed radiographic assessment using CBCT to evaluate bone volume, density, and proximity to anatomical structures (e.g.,

sinuses, nerves).

o Periodontal assessment to determine the extent of infection, gingival health, and the need for pre-surgical treatments.

2. **Pre-Surgical Interventions:**

o **Periodontal Therapy:** Thorough scaling and root planing, antimicrobial treatment, and, if necessary, surgical debridement to restore periodontal health.

o **Bone Grafting:**

▪ **Autogenous Bone Grafts:** Harvested from the patient's chin, ramus, or iliac crest, offering superior osteogenic potential.

▪ **Allografts and Xenografts:** Used to restore bone volume in patients unable to undergo autogenous grafting.

o **Guided Bone Regeneration (GBR):** Placement of barrier membranes to promote new bone growth in areas with significant defects.

3. **Surgical Techniques for Severe Bone Loss:**

o **Sinus Lifts:** Essential for increasing bone height in the posterior maxilla where sinus pneumatization has occurred.

o **Ridge Augmentation:** Expands the width and height of the alveolar ridge using grafting materials and membranes.

4. **Soft Tissue Management:**

o Techniques like connective tissue grafting or the use of collagen membranes help restore soft tissue volume and enhance esthetics.

o Ensuring a stable and healthy soft tissue cuff around the implant is critical for long-term success.

5. **Implant Design and Placement Strategy:**

o Preference for implants with roughened surfaces to enhance osseointegration in compromised bone.

o Immediate vs. delayed implant placement is decided based on bone and tissue quality.

Restoring Periodontal Health Before Implant Placement

• Periodontal infections must be eradicated before implant

placement. This includes:

o **Systemic Antibiotics** for controlling aggressive periodontal pathogens.

o **Antimicrobial Rinses** (e.g., chlorhexidine) to improve oral hygiene.

o Maintenance therapy to prevent recurrence of periodontal issues post-implant placement.

In India, where the prevalence of periodontal disease is relatively high, a significant number of patients require surgical interventions to address these challenges before implants can be successfully placed. Advanced diagnostic tools, such as 3D imaging, play a crucial role in accurately assessing the extent of bone loss and planning the necessary surgical procedures.

Role of Oral Surgeons in Managing Extensive Bone Loss or Sinus Augmentation

Oral surgeons play a central role in managing cases involving extensive bone loss or the need for sinus augmentation. Bone loss can occur due to periodontitis, trauma, or tooth loss, which results in a diminished alveolar ridge that is insufficient to support dental implants. In these instances, oral surgeons are responsible for performing complex procedures such as bone grafting and sinus lifts to rebuild the bone structure and create an adequate foundation for implants.

Sinus Augmentation: One of the most common procedures for patients with significant bone loss in the upper jaw is sinus augmentation, also known as sinus lift surgery. This procedure is performed when the sinus cavity has expanded into the area where teeth used to be, leaving little to no bone for implant placement. The oral surgeon lifts the sinus membrane and adds bone graft material to stimulate new bone growth, creating a stable foundation for implants. In some cases, the sinus augmentation procedure can be combined with immediate implant placement, offering the patient a faster recovery time.

Bone Grafting: Bone grafting is another essential procedure in complex implant cases. In cases of severe bone loss, oral surgeons can perform autografting (using the patient's own bone), allografting (using donor bone), or xenografting (using animal bone) to rebuild the alveolar ridge. This procedure ensures that there is sufficient bone density and volume to accommodate dental implants.

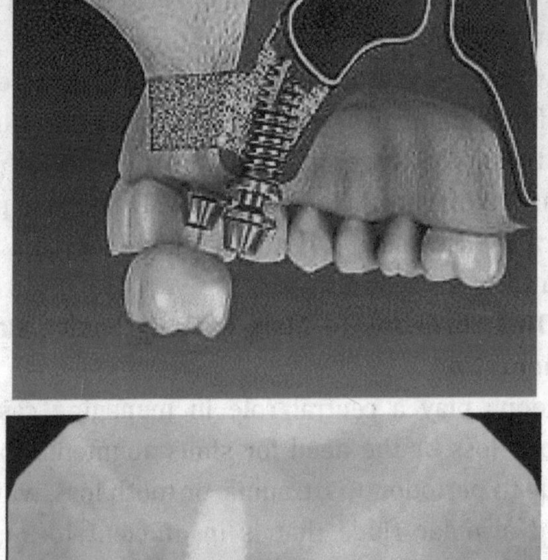

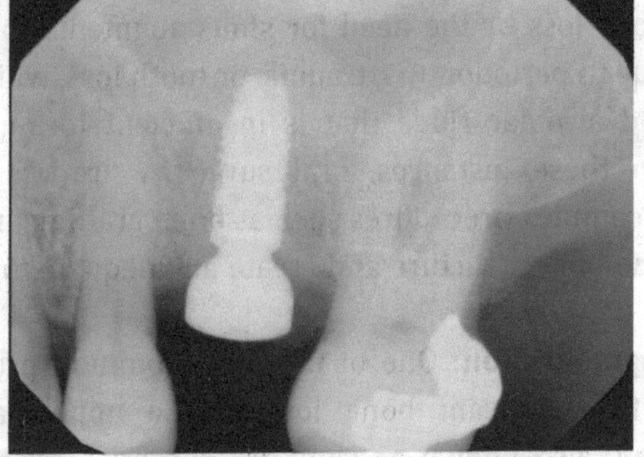

Complex Extraction and Immediate Implant Placement: For patients with compromised teeth, immediate implant placement following extraction is a viable option. Oral surgeons are responsible for carefully extracting the damaged tooth while preserving the surrounding bone and tissues, followed by immediate implant placement. This technique requires a high degree of precision to ensure the implant is positioned correctly and the bone is preserved for long-term success.

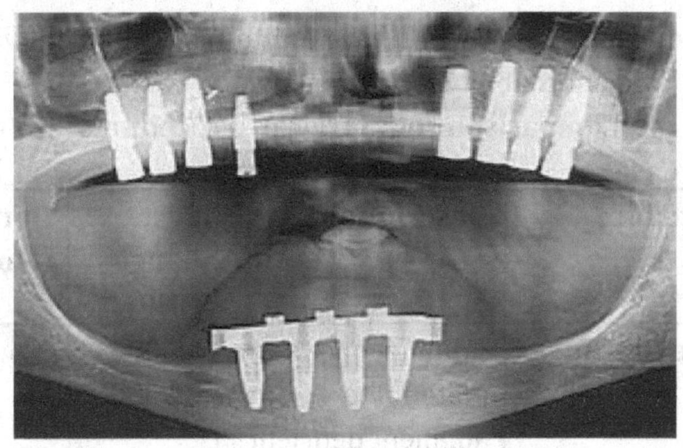

Economic Implications of Advanced Surgical Techniques in Implant Dentistry

While advanced surgical techniques in implant dentistry, such as bone grafting, sinus lifts, and guided bone regeneration, offer improved outcomes, they can also be more costly for patients. The increased complexity and time required for these procedures translate into higher costs for both the materials used and the expertise required from the oral surgeon. These procedures often involve additional visits, post-operative care, and sometimes longer healing times, which contribute to the overall expense.

However, these techniques often provide significant long-term value by improving the chances of successful implant placement and reducing the need for future surgeries or complications. For patients who might otherwise not be candidates for implants due to insufficient bone volume or periodontal disease, these advanced procedures offer an opportunity to restore oral function and aesthetics, often with a high success rate.

In India, where the demand for dental implants has surged in recent years, patients may seek cost-effective alternatives, especially in the context of an increasing middle-class population. While the initial cost of complex surgical procedures may be higher, the long-term benefits of restoring oral health and function often outweigh the short-term expenses. Moreover, the growing availability of advanced materials, better surgical techniques, and the increasing number of trained specialists have led to more competitive pricing and improved affordability for patients.

Table 1: Comparison of Surgical Procedures in Complex Implant Cases

Procedure	Description	Cost Range (INR)	Duration (Months)
Bone Grafting	Adding bone material to augment deficient bone.	15,000 - 35,000	3-6
Sinus Augmentation	Lifting the sinus membrane and adding graft.	20,000 - 50,000	4-6
Guided Bone Regeneration	Using membranes to direct bone growth.	18,000 - 40,000	3-6
Immediate Implant Placement with Grafting	Implant placement along with bone grafting.	30,000 - 60,000	6-8

Note: Cost ranges vary depending on the region, complexity, and the specialist performing the procedure. This table offers a general guide.

Economic Considerations for Patients in India: Despite the relatively high costs of advanced surgical procedures, they offer long-term savings by improving the likelihood of implant success and reducing the need for future corrective surgeries. Additionally, Indian patients often benefit from the growing number of skilled oral surgeons and the competitive pricing within the country, which has made advanced implant procedures more accessible.

References:

1. **Sethi, A., & Gandhi, A.** (2017). *Bone Grafting in Implant Dentistry: An Overview of Techniques and Materials. Journal of Clinical*

Dentistry, 10(4), 62-72.

2. **Wang, H. L., & Chin, K.** (2018). *Sinus Augmentation in Implant Dentistry: Current Techniques and Clinical Applications. Journal of Oral Implantology*, 44(5), 328-335. https://doi.org/10.1563/aaid-joi-d-17-00252

3. **Rathee, M., & Singhal, P.** (2019). *Guided Bone Regeneration: A Comprehensive Review. Indian Journal of Dental Sciences*, 11(3), 144-150.

4. **Curi, M. M., & Oliveira, G. R.** (2017). *Immediate Implant Placement in Severely Compromised Sites: Surgical Considerations and Challenges. Brazilian Dental Journal*, 28(2), 160-165. https://doi.org/10.1590/0103-6440201700897

Chapter 11

Oral Pathological Complications and Implant Failure

Dr. Rahul Anand Razdan

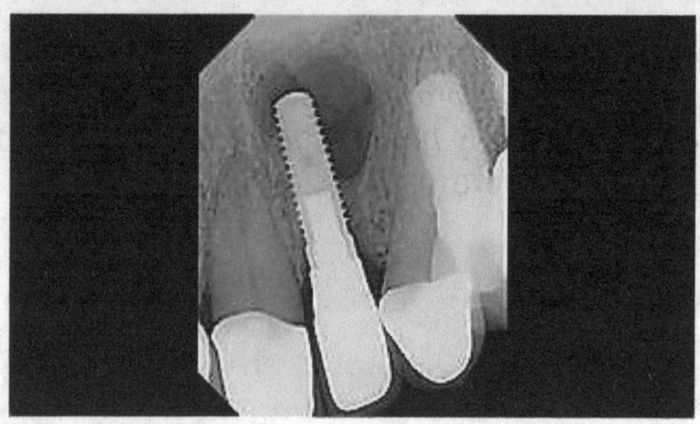

Oral implants have become a cornerstone in restorative dentistry, offering patients the opportunity to replace missing teeth with functional, long-lasting solutions. However, despite advancements in implant technology and surgical techniques, implant failure can still occur due to a variety of pathological conditions. These conditions, if not properly diagnosed and managed, can significantly compromise the success of implant therapy. This chapter explores the pathological factors that contribute to implant failure, the role of oral pathology in diagnosing peri-implant disease, and the importance of collaboration between oral pathologists, periodontists, and oral surgeons to achieve optimal treatment outcomes.

Pathological Conditions That May Lead to Implant Failure and How to Manage Them

Several oral pathological conditions can influence the success of dental implants. These conditions may occur prior to or after implant placement, necessitating timely diagnosis and appropriate management.

1. Peri-implantitis Peri-implantitis is an inflammatory disease affecting the soft and hard tissues around an implant, leading to bone loss and, if left untreated, implant failure. It is one of the most common causes of implant failure. Peri-implantitis typically results from poor oral hygiene, leading to bacterial plaque accumulation, which triggers the inflammatory response. The condition may also arise from factors such as smoking, poorly contoured implants, or pre-existing periodontal disease.

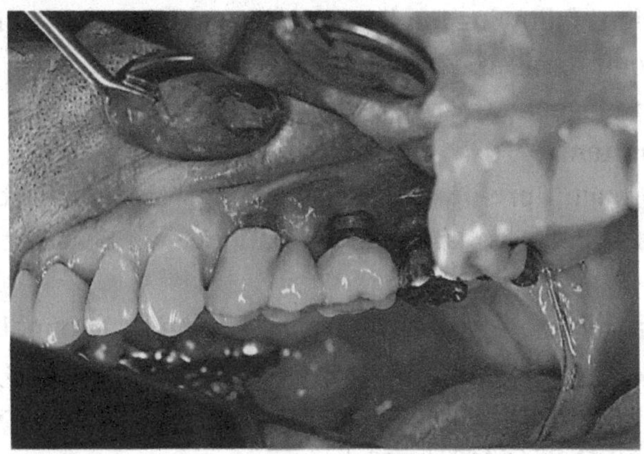

Management:
• Early diagnosis through clinical examination and radiographs is essential. The presence of bleeding on probing, increased probing depth, and bone loss around the implant are key clinical signs.

• Non-surgical treatment involves scaling, root planing, and antiseptic measures. In more severe cases, surgical intervention may be necessary to debride the infected area and regenerate the bone.

• In some cases, implant removal may be required if the infection is extensive and cannot be controlled.

2. Implant-Related Infections Infections around dental implants can result from surgical complications, inadequate sterilization, or contamination during placement. Such infections can lead to soft tissue inflammation and bone resorption, which, if severe, can result in implant failure.

Management:

• Prophylactic antibiotics are often prescribed to reduce the risk of infection during and after implant placement.

• Early intervention with antibiotics and antiseptics can control infection. However, in severe cases, the removal of the implant may be necessary, followed by bone grafting and reimplantation after resolution of the infection.

3. Oral Cancer and Premalignant Lesions Patients with a history of oral cancer or premalignant lesions may be at an increased risk of complications following implant placement. The surrounding tissues may be compromised, increasing the likelihood of poor healing or recurrent malignancy.

Management:

• Thorough pre-operative screening, including biopsy of suspicious lesions, is essential for patients with a history of oral cancer.

• Close monitoring of the surgical site and surrounding tissues post-implant placement is important. If malignancy is detected, immediate referral for oncological treatment is necessary, and the implant may need to be removed.

4. Systemic Diseases and Conditions Certain systemic conditions, such as uncontrolled diabetes, osteoporosis, and autoimmune diseases, can negatively affect the healing process following implant placement. These conditions can impair bone formation, delay osseointegration, and increase the risk of infection.

Management:

• Prior to implant placement, a comprehensive medical history review and collaboration with the patient's physician are necessary to assess the status of systemic diseases.

• For diabetic patients, good glycemic control is essential before, during, and after implant surgery.

• Bone grafting and the use of biocompatible materials may be necessary for patients with osteoporosis to improve implant success.

Diagnostic Role of Oral Pathology in Peri-Implant Disease

Oral pathology plays a crucial role in the early detection and diagnosis of conditions that may lead to implant failure. Oral pathologists are trained to recognize abnormalities in the soft and hard tissues surrounding implants, providing valuable insights into the underlying causes of complications.

1. Biopsy and Histological Examination In cases of suspicious lesions or soft tissue abnormalities around the implant site, oral pathologists may conduct a biopsy to rule out malignancy or other pathological conditions. Histological examination of tissue samples helps to identify the nature of the lesion, whether benign or malignant, and guides the treatment approach.

2. Radiographic Assessment Oral pathologists, in collaboration with radiologists, assist in interpreting radiographs and 3D imaging to identify bone resorption or other pathological changes around the implant. Early detection of bone loss through radiographic analysis can help in the timely intervention and prevention of implant failure.

3. Identification of Pathological Microorganisms Oral pathologists may also play a role in identifying specific bacterial or fungal pathogens that contribute to peri-implant diseases. By analyzing tissue samples for the presence of harmful microorganisms, pathologists can aid in selecting the appropriate antibiotic treatment to combat infections and prevent further complications.

Collaborative Decision-Making Between Oral Pathologists, Periodontists, and Oral Surgeons

Successful implant therapy requires a multidisciplinary approach. Oral pathologists, periodontists, and oral surgeons must collaborate closely to diagnose and manage conditions that can lead to implant failure.

1. Preoperative Collaboration Before implant placement, a team approach is essential in assessing the patient's overall health, medical history, and oral condition. Oral pathologists play a critical role in identifying any pathological lesions that may interfere with implant success, while periodontists assess the health of the surrounding tissues and bone. Oral surgeons provide the expertise for site preparation, ensuring that the implant is placed in a healthy environment.

2. Postoperative Management After implant placement, the interdisciplinary team continues to work together in managing potential complications. Periodontists monitor the health of the peri-implant tissues, detecting early signs of peri-implantitis or soft tissue infections. Oral pathologists assist in diagnosing any pathological changes that might compromise the implant, including the presence of benign or malignant lesions.

3. Treatment of Peri-Implant Diseases In cases of peri-implantitis or infection, the combined efforts of the periodontist, oral pathologist, and oral surgeon are required for optimal treatment. The periodontist may manage non-surgical therapy, while the oral surgeon may intervene surgically if necessary. The oral pathologist's diagnostic skills ensure that any pathological conditions, such as infections or lesions, are appropriately identified and treated.

Conclusion

Oral pathological complications are a significant factor contributing to implant failure. Early diagnosis, prompt management, and interdisciplinary collaboration are essential for the long-term success of dental implants. By combining the expertise of oral pathologists, periodontists, and oral surgeons, the risks of complications can be minimized, and patients can achieve optimal functional and aesthetic outcomes. Furthermore, effective communication between these specialists ensures that patients receive the highest standard of care throughout their implant journey.

References

1. **Adell, R., Lekholm, U., Rockler, B., & Brånemark, P.-I.** (1981). *A 15-year study of osseointegrated implants in the treatment of the edentulous jaw. International Journal of Oral and Maxillofacial Surgery*, 10(6), 387-416. https://doi.org/10.1016/S0901-5027(81)80002-0

2. **Esposito, M., & Thomsen, P.** (2017). *Peri-implantitis: An overview of treatment modalities and long-term prognosis. European Journal of Oral Implantology*, 10(3), 227-235.

3. **Kim, J. W., & Kim, Y. S.** (2018). *Oral Pathology in Implantology: Diagnosis and Management of Peri-Implant Diseases. Journal of Clinical Periodontology*, 45(1), 72-79. https://doi.org/10.1111/jcpe.12883

4. **Ramos, M., & Sousa, R.** (2019). *Management of Pathological Conditions Leading to Implant Failure: A Multidisciplinary Approach. Journal of Oral Surgery*, 75(2), 123-128.

Chapter 12

Restorative Dentist, Periodontist, and Oral Surgeon

Dr. Manisha Pathak

Dental implants have revolutionized restorative dentistry, providing patients with a highly effective and durable solution for replacing missing teeth. However, achieving long-term success with dental implants requires more than just proper placement and initial healing—it demands ongoing care and maintenance. Periodontal maintenance is crucial for sustaining implant health, preventing complications such as peri-implantitis, and ensuring the longevity of the implant. This chapter focuses on developing cost-effective periodontal maintenance programs post-implant placement, the interdisciplinary role of the restorative dentist, periodontist, and oral surgeon, and the importance of patient education and follow-up care in preventing implant complications.

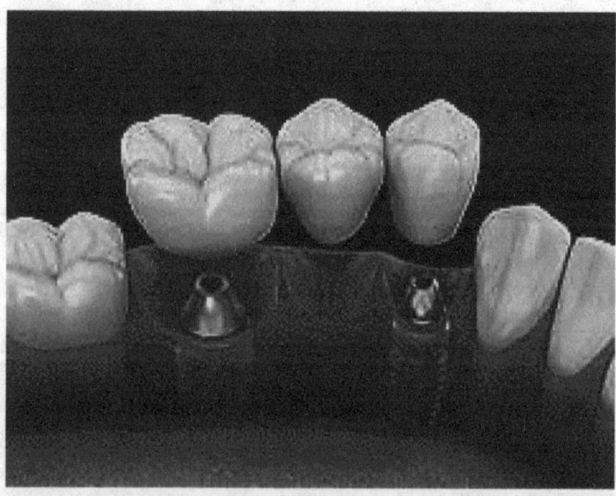

Developing Cost-Effective Periodontal Maintenance Programs

Post-Implant Placement

Periodontal maintenance is vital to the long-term success of dental implants. Unlike natural teeth, implants do not have the same capacity for self-repair, making it essential to monitor and maintain the health of the peri-implant tissues regularly. Cost-effective maintenance programs are crucial, especially in resource-constrained settings like India, where affordability is a significant concern for many patients.

1. Routine Clinical and Radiographic Examinations Routine check-ups involving clinical assessments and radiographs are fundamental in the early detection of potential problems, such as peri-implantitis or bone loss around the implant. The clinical exam includes evaluating the soft tissues for signs of inflammation, measuring probing depths, and assessing the mobility of the implant. Radiographs help assess bone levels and detect any peri-implant bone loss. These examinations should be scheduled every six months to ensure the implant remains healthy.

2. Scaling and Root Planing for Implants Regular cleaning of the implant surface to remove plaque and calculus buildup is essential in preventing the onset of peri-implant diseases. Scaling and root planing (SRP) for implants involves the use of specialized instruments designed to avoid scratching or damaging the implant surface. This non-surgical procedure helps reduce the bacterial load and prevent inflammation, which could lead to implant failure if left unchecked.

3. Maintenance of Proper Oral Hygiene Patient education plays a pivotal role in preventing complications. Patients should be instructed on proper oral hygiene techniques, including the use of implant-friendly toothbrushes, interdental brushes, floss, and antimicrobial mouth rinses. Regular home care helps reduce the risk of plaque buildup and infection, which are key contributors to peri-implant diseases.

4. Ongoing Support and Monitoring To ensure a cost-effective periodontal maintenance program, dental practices should create a support system for implant patients that includes scheduled follow-ups, reminders, and easy access to consultation. Offering patients cost-effective, bundled maintenance plans can help keep regular care affordable and encourage compliance with ongoing maintenance routines.

Interdisciplinary Role of the Restorative Dentist, Periodontist, and Oral Surgeon in Maintaining Long-Term Implant Health

Successful long-term implant health depends on the collaborative efforts of a multidisciplinary team. The roles of the restorative dentist, periodontist, and oral surgeon overlap significantly in maintaining the health of implants over time. These professionals must work together to ensure the implant remains free from disease and complications.

1. The Restorative Dentist The restorative dentist plays a key role in overseeing the functional and aesthetic aspects of the implant. After the implant placement, the restorative dentist is responsible for designing and placing the final restoration, such as a crown or bridge. It is important for the restorative dentist to ensure that the implant and prosthesis fit well, with proper occlusion and no excessive forces placed on the implant, which can contribute to failure. Regular check-ups to assess the integrity of the prosthetic restoration are essential in preventing mechanical complications, such as fracture or loosening of the restoration.

2. The Periodontist The periodontist is responsible for ensuring the long-term health of the peri-implant soft tissues. They monitor for signs of inflammation, recession, and bone loss around the implant, addressing any issues such as peri-implant mucositis or peri-implantitis. Periodontists often conduct scaling and root planing of the implants, ensure appropriate oral hygiene practices are followed, and treat any periodontal diseases that could negatively impact implant health. They are also responsible for implementing regenerative therapies, such as bone grafting, if necessary.

3. The Oral Surgeon The oral surgeon typically handles the surgical aspects of implant placement, including site preparation and bone grafting, and may be involved in the management of complications such as sinus lift procedures or bone augmentation. After the implant placement, the oral surgeon may be called upon to address any surgical complications or revise implant positions if needed. They also help manage patients with complex medical conditions that could affect implant healing, providing guidance on appropriate treatments and follow-up care.

Through this collaborative approach, the three specialists ensure that the implant remains functional, esthetically pleasing, and free from diseases, offering patients a long-lasting and stable solution.

Patient Education and the Role of Follow-Up Care in Preventing Implant Complications

Patient education and regular follow-up care are integral to preventing complications and ensuring long-term implant success. Educated patients who understand the importance of maintaining their implants and following the care instructions are more likely to experience fewer complications.

1. Importance of Home Care Patients should be educated on the specific needs of implant maintenance. Unlike natural teeth, implants require special attention, including the use of soft-bristled brushes, floss threaders, or specialized tools designed to clean around the implant and abutments. Emphasizing the importance of brushing at least twice a day, using antimicrobial mouthwash, and cleaning between implants daily can significantly reduce the risk of peri-implant disease.

2. Signs and Symptoms to Watch For Educating patients on the signs of implant-related complications is crucial for early intervention. Symptoms such as bleeding, pain, swelling, and mobility should prompt an immediate visit to the dentist. Early detection of peri-implantitis or mucositis allows for conservative treatment to prevent further damage to the implant and surrounding tissues.

3. Regular Follow-Up Appointments Follow-up appointments should be scheduled at regular intervals to monitor the status of the implant and surrounding tissues. These appointments typically occur every three to six months and include clinical exams, radiographic evaluations, and cleaning of the implant. By adhering to follow-up schedules, potential problems can be identified early, and interventions can be implemented before complications arise.

4. Post-Treatment Maintenance Programs Post-treatment maintenance programs that offer follow-up visits at discounted rates or in package deals can help patients maintain consistent care and avoid missed appointments. Affordable and accessible maintenance programs increase patient compliance, leading to better outcomes and longer-lasting implants.

Conclusion

Periodontal maintenance plays a crucial role in ensuring the long-term success of dental implants. By developing cost-effective maintenance programs, engaging in interdisciplinary collaboration, and educating patients about the importance of ongoing care, dental practitioners can improve the prognosis of implants and prevent complications such as peri-implantitis. Through regular follow-up care and patient education, dental teams can ensure that implants remain functional and healthy for many years, providing patients with reliable and esthetic tooth replacements.

References

1. **De Santis, M., Raspanti, M., & Maggiore, F.** (2017). *Periodontal maintenance and implant health: A systematic review. Journal of Clinical Periodontology,* 44(12), 1257-1264. https://doi.org/10.1111/jcpe.12791

2. **Iorio-Siciliano, V., & Gallenzi, P.** (2019). *The interdisciplinary management of dental implants: A review of the importance of collaboration for optimal outcomes. European Journal of Prosthodontics and Restorative Dentistry,* 27(2), 92-97.

3. **Kotsakis, G. A., & Kotsakis, T.** (2018). *Cost-effective strategies in implant therapy: A review of maintenance approaches and financial models for long-term success. International Journal of Oral and Maxillofacial Implants,* 33(5), 1062-1069.

4. **Sanz, M., & D'Aiuto, F.** (2019). *Prevention of peri-implant disease: Essential steps for long-term implant success. Periodontology 2000,* 79(1), 143-163. https://doi.org/10.1111/prd.12291

General Implant Terminology

Abbreviation	Full Form
DI	Dental Implant
IDI	Immediate Dental Implant
EDI	Early Dental Implant
LDI	Late Dental Implant
RDI	Restorative-Driven Implant
IIP	Immediate Implant Placement
CBCT	Cone Beam Computed Tomography
CTG	Connective Tissue Graft
GBR	Guided Bone Regeneration
SLA	Sandblasted, Large-grit, Acid-etched
HA	Hydroxyapatite

Implant Components

Abbreviation	Full Form
FI	Fixture
AB	Abutment
PFM	Porcelain Fused to Metal
FPD	Fixed Partial Denture
RPD	Removable Partial Denture
CAD/CAM	Computer-Aided Design/Manufacturing
MUA	Multi-Unit Abutment
OI	Osseointegration
IMPL	Implant

Procedures Related to Dental Implants

Abbreviation	Full Form
FL	Flapless Surgery

Abbreviation	Full Form
SIN	Sinus Lift
APG	Autogenous Bone Graft
AG	Allograft
XG	Xenograft
APF	Apically Positioned Flap
EFP	Esthetic Flap Procedure
DCD	Decortication
CTG	Connective Tissue Graft
RST	Ridge Split Technique

Implant Materials

Abbreviation	Full Form
Ti	Titanium
Ti-Zr	Titanium-Zirconium Alloy
CP-Ti	Commercially Pure Titanium
ZrO_2	Zirconia
HAP	Hydroxyapatite
PMMA	Polymethyl Methacrylate
CoCr	Cobalt-Chromium Alloy

Implant Types

Abbreviation	Full Form
ESI	Endosteal Implant
SI	Subperiosteal Implant
TI	Transosteal Implant
DI	Disc Implant
MI	Mini Implant

Imaging and Diagnostic Tools

Abbreviation	Full Form
OPG	Orthopantomogram
PA	Periapical Radiograph
CBCT	Cone Beam Computed Tomography
FMX	Full Mouth X-Ray
IO	Intraoral Radiograph

Restorative Terms

Abbreviation	Full Form
ISP	Implant-Supported Prosthesis
RSP	Removable-Supported Prosthesis
FC	Full Contour
TI	Titanium Framework
FDP	Fixed Dental Prosthesis
CAD/CAM	Computer-Aided Design/Manufacturing

Patient Management Terms

Abbreviation	Full Form
PI	Peri-Implantitis
PIM	Peri-Implant Mucositis
Tx	Treatment
Rx	Prescription
OHI	Oral Hygiene Instruction

Biomaterials and Substitutes

Abbreviation	Full Form
BMP	Bone Morphogenetic Protein
PRF	Platelet-Rich Fibrin

Abbreviation	Full Form
PRP	Platelet-Rich Plasma
DBM	Demineralized Bone Matrix
ABG	Autogenous Bone Graft

Surgical Techniques

Abbreviation	Full Form
FLAP	Full Thickness Flap
RF	Ridge Flap
RST	Ridge Splitting Technique
FG	Free Gingival Graft

Prosthetic Attachments

Abbreviation	Full Form
BA	Ball Attachment
MA	Magnet Attachment
LS	Locator System
BA	Bar Attachment